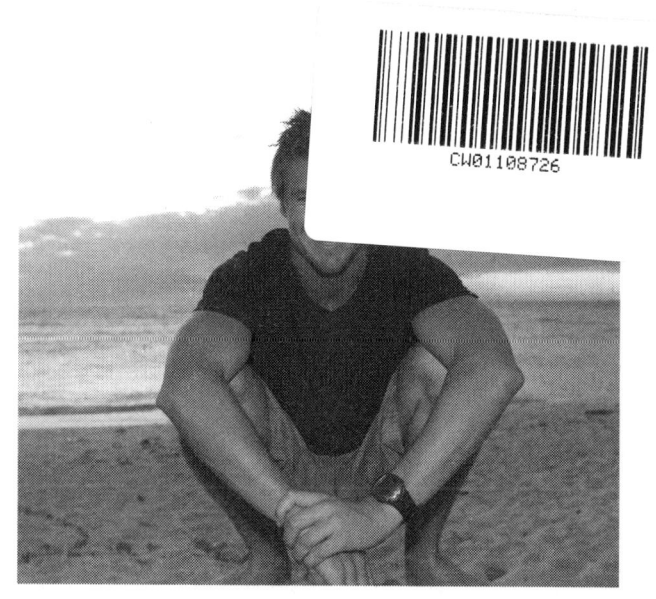

Matt Griggs was born in 1976 into a beach-loving family and grew up in the surfing heartland of Cronulla in the south of Sydney. He competed around the world as a professional surfer before retiring in 1999 to work as a staff writer for *Tracks* magazine. His first book, *Surfers*, was published in 2002. Since 2003 he has worked as the 'Pit Boss' for Rip Curl's international surf team.

# a wave away

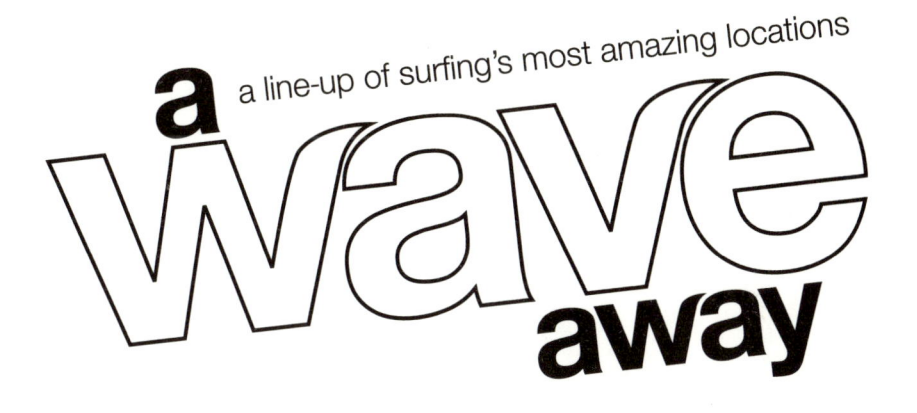

a line-up of surfing's most amazing locations

## MATT GRIGGS

*To Colin*
*Happy 50th birthday*
*love from*
*Ann + Steve*
*x*

**Harper**Sports
An imprint of HarperCollins*Publishers*

**Harper***Sports*
An imprint of HarperCollins*Publishers*, Australia

First published in Australia in 2008
by HarperCollins*Publishers* Australia Pty Limited
ABN 36 009 913 517
www.harpercollins.com.au

Copyright © Matt Griggs 2008

The right of Matt Griggs to be identified as the author of this work has been asserted by him under the *Copyright Amendment (Moral Rights) Act 2000*.

This work is copyright.
Apart from any use as permitted under the *Copyright Act 1968*, no part may be reproduced, copied, scanned, stored in a retrieval system, recorded, or transmitted, in any form or by any means, without the prior written permission of the publisher.

**HarperCollins***Publishers*
25 Ryde Road, Pymble, Sydney NSW 2073, Australia
31 View Road, Glenfield, Auckland 10, New Zealand
1-A, Hamilton House, Connaught Place, New Delhi – 110 001, India
77–85 Fulham Palace Road, London W6 8JB, United Kingdom
2 Bloor Street East, 20th floor, Toronto, Ontario M4W 1A8, Canada
10 East 53rd Street, New York NY 10022, USA

National Library of Australia Cataloguing-in-Publication data:

Griggs, Matt.
  A wave away: a line-up of surfing's most amazing locations / Matt Griggs
  ISBN: 978 0 7322 8638 5 (pbk.).
  Surfing. Surfers.
797.32

Cover design by Matt Stanton
Front cover photograph by Jon Frank
Back cover photographs: girls by Ted Grambeau; surfer by Matt Kelson;
car by Ted Grambeau; lighthouse by Jon Frank
Internal photos courtesy of Shutterstock except where otherwise credited.
Typeset in 10.5/18pt Giovanni Book by Helen Beard, ECJ Australia Pty Limited
Printed and bound in Australia by Griffin Press
70gsm Classic used by HarperCollins*Publishers* is a natural, recyclable product made from wood grown in sustainable forests. The manufacturing processes conform to the environmental regulations in the country of origin, Finland.

7 6 5 4 3 2 1    08 09 10 11 12

*I want to dedicate this book to the natural beauty
of the world and those who preserve it.*

# CONTENTS

| | |
|---:|---:|
| Introduction | ix |
| Shock Waves | 1 |
| Stars and Strife | 17 |
| South of … Opportunity | 45 |
| King Teahupoo's Ghost | 53 |
| The New Archipelago | 61 |
| Wretches in Paradise | 68 |
| Native Mysteries | 76 |
| The Southern Cross Over | 84 |
| 17,508 | 104 |
| Beyond Cloud Nine | 124 |
| Mayhem and Mama-San | 132 |
| Lionise | 147 |
| The Business Was Survival | 166 |
| Place d'Afrique | 172 |
| Living the Mirage | 178 |
| The Long Walk | 191 |
| Beneath a Monotone Sky | 206 |
| … And Then the Wind Stopped | 213 |
| Vive le Oui | 223 |
| From ETA to Eucalpyt | 234 |
| Nordic Fresh | 241 |
| Corridor of Contrast | 250 |
| Buenos Dias | 261 |
| Meat in the Sandwich | 266 |
| Jungle Booty | 269 |
| The Sands of All Time | 280 |

## introduction
# THE EDGE OF THE WORLD

Standing at the edge of the world I can see it all: the places I've been, the few places yet to come. They are all there, where most dreams start — over the horizon. It's July 2007, and I'm at the Cape of Good Hope.

Standing here, it really feels as if you're on earth's last bridge, casting your eyes over infinity, gazing into possibilities. There's nothing between you and Antarctica — nothing, except a whole lot of ocean.

On one side the Atlantic is furious, lashing winds whipping white horses into thirty-foot waves, sending sea-spray up the cliffs, carrying the smell of life and death. On the other side, the Indian Ocean is in quiet meditation. The strong winds here are heading in the same direction as the swell — offshore — leaving the coastline quiet. You can't help but look back and forth at the two oceans, two moods, two different temperature zones, thirty-foot waves and two-foot waves. A stubborn headland stands between them as if it is holding back a fight. All the elements of nature don't just meet here; they collide.

Behind me — as is their habit — a baboon has stolen some food from a tourist's grasp. She panics. In the reserve, zebras roam, springbok triple jump with grace through the thick salt air and ostriches peck away at the brush, stopping occasionally to look at the view. There is a change in the weather — a common occurrence here — and they are the first to notice it. The wind becomes so strong that even the baboons are starting to react. Menacing dark clouds gather; they have no shape, no extremities. The sky is just black. You can see the ghosts of years of shipwrecks turning in their grave. The stubborn brush is the only thing that doesn't run for shelter; it's seen it all before. Car doors close, windows are wound, engines start. Below the headland a surfer is running in the other direction — past the baboons, over the top of the brush and into the ocean.

I smile in recognition of his impulse. I am a person who is inspired by the elements of nature, who enjoys connecting with the raw power and whose heartbeat increases with excitement when nature turns on a show. I look at the rocks below, which, in bad weather, have been the end-point for many journeys. The lighthouse reminds me that sometimes humans need help when they come to this place.

For me, this place was the halfway point in the writing of this book — the infinite horizon was inspiring and its perspective offered some reflection.

I've lived on this edge constantly, chasing this weather at times, and have evolved like the stubborn brush that clings to most coastlines. It may not be literally the edge of the world here, but when you are put in a position like this, a landscape like this, you can definitely imagine it.

When it comes to being in the right position, I have led a fortunate life. I travel around the world as 'Pit Boss' for surfing giant Rip Curl, coaching, mentoring, mothering, fathering and managing the affairs of our team on the World Championship Tour. Sometimes it seems like the hardest job in the world and sometimes I can't believe I get paid to do it. I video the team members surfing, take notes of their heats, tinker with technique, mould, manoeuvre, manufacture and measure mental mindsets, constantly looking for improvement in their performance and daily lives. We start in Australia, go through the Pacific (Tahiti and Fiji), then to South Africa, Japan, California, Brazil, Europe, Hawaii ... We find waves, experience the culture and taste the local delights. We know how to pack in one minute flat; we know flight connections and flight numbers like our own phone numbers; we know the best restaurants, the best surf breaks — and pages in our passports disappear like notes in our wallets. We know how to say 'where/what/who and how' in every coastal language; we know which check-in lady is more likely to charge excess; and we know, by the feel of the air, what weather will dawn. This is the peak of life's experiences — the opportunity to have an amazing view of the world and the people who inhabit it.

I'll never forget the phone call from my former action sports publisher at *Tracks*, Neil Ridgway, who was then the International Marketing Director for Rip Curl. 'I'm creating this position to support our surfers on the World Championship Tour ... Are you interested?' I clasped my hand around the phone and screamed, 'Wooooooooooooooo!' Then I cleared my throat, looked up at the *Tracks* building where I'd just spent all night enduring another deadline, and said, 'Go on.' I had found my calling — or, since a job like this didn't exist, it had found me.

Working with people like Mick Fanning and our support network means I am surrounded by some forward-thinking minds. These are people who are willing to trade comfort for experience, to evolve as people every day, to ask questions and look for answers. They approach life head-on. When you pack that mindset in your travel bag, it is amazing the experiences you can have.

I have the unique position of having access to the world's best surfers and the places they venture, not just on the World Championship Tour, but also on what Rip Curl calls 'The Search', which, combined with our World Tour stops, has taken us through Indonesia, Micronesia, wider Africa, New Zealand and Morocco. Sometimes, since I'm already on the road, I take time to visit another country, like Israel or Ireland, before heading to the next tour spot. When I go home, even if only for a week, I get asked a lot of questions about the event, so I never feel as if I have a break from it. So I've learned to sometimes stay away, to venture into new worlds where I can ask the questions.

My current team are Mick Fanning, Taylor Knox, Pancho Sullivan, Ben Dunn and Ricky Basnett, but guys like Nathan Hedge and members of the greater surfing community also find their way into the following stories. We have often been to the places we visit not just once, but sometimes up to fifteen times. So we have developed friendships, families, and a deeper understanding of what is beyond the guy stamping our passports.

I hadn't written much since the publication of *Surfers* in 2002, instead choosing to focus on my new job. But the familiar signs were there. If I don't write, my speech starts to become unnecessarily creative, my emails turn into poems or short stories and my friends call me weird. Plus, as I was going to so many amazing places full of interesting people, I had to agree: it was time to write again. So along came my new project: *A Wave Away*. It became the creative culmination of all this experience; the true test of the survival of the fittest, where only the best stories made the grade. Writing this book also brought me closer to the places to which we had travelled. To write about a place, you have to understand it, you have to speak to interesting people, share their passion, their fears and their lives. You have to look beyond the words and feel the emotion. I put myself in some challenging situations and this really brought me closer to whatever life force governs our shared existence.

I looked a little deeper and cast my net a little wider. I travelled to some new places, searching for unique experiences, trying to connect to different cultures — whether it was people bitten by sharks, ravaged by AIDS, swallowed by forty-foot waves, chasing world titles, or watching the sun going down over the Mediterranean at dusk.

These are experiences we hear of, but don't often live through ourselves — things we fear, things that inspire us, that sadden us, excite us ... the gaps between life and death, the wondering what is out there, beyond the edge of the world and over the horizon. This book is a modest attempt to describe these experiences and feelings through the eyes and ears of a travelling Pit Boss. It is written by someone who is fascinated by humans and inspired by the heartbeat of life, observing and recording from the edge of the world a culture that really is a wave away, and hopefully bringing the horizon to you every time you turn a page.

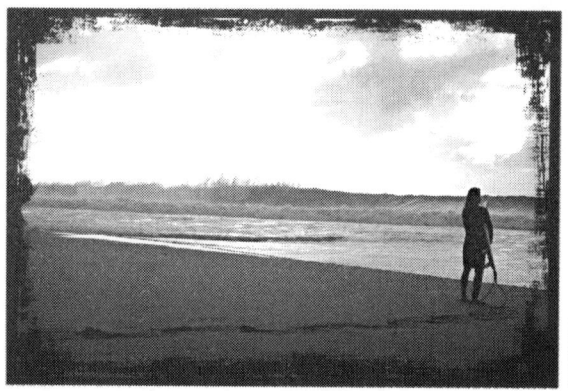

# SHOCK WAVES
## HAWAII

'Tall and proud as a mountain, carved by the hands of man ... the honour from which it stands ... is held steadfast as a reminder of the native people and the inherent rights which it represents ...'

Carved from a huge hardwood tree, the big *titu* head at Rocky Point has seen it all — from the Polynesian ancestors to the white settlers; from the disintegration of the traditional monarchical system to the annexation by the United States; from hardwood surfboards negotiating waves like poetry, to fibreglass thrusters riding waves and stardom. It may be one of the world's youngest landmasses, but surfing in Hawaii seems to be as ancient as the ocean itself and, like the ocean, only partly understood.

There are entries in Captain James Cook's logs of people riding waves when he first threw anchor in 1778. 'The boldness and address, with which we saw them perform these difficult and dangerous manoeuvres, was altogether astonishing, and is scarcely to be credited.' There are even detailed pictures of Hawaiians riding their wooden planks in cave drawings centuries old. It was a simple life then. Like most Polynesians, they lived off and on the water. It gave life, it taught life, it saved lives, it took lives. These days, many people are attracted to the tropical pleasures of Hawaii and although you have to look hard to find the traditional culture in its physical form, there is an aloha spirit everywhere you can almost feel and touch. From the waves, to the volcanic mountains, to the odd big *titu* head voicing a past and welcoming a future, the aloha spirit is still alive.

## THESE COLOURS DON'T FADE, THESE ROOTS WON'T DIE

His name was Ross; he was a softly spoken full-blooded Polynesian who just oozed flow. But beneath the rhythm wrestled a story of a past beyond his own. He lived on Oahu's east side, about an hour's drive from the North Shore in a large town called Kaneohe. Ross had his own green-keeping business and was a very keen surfer. Whether it was howling cross shore at Sunset Point, or maxing at Waimea, Ross was out there.

One day, he was pulled over by the police on his way back home. They had noticed that his number plates weren't standard USA/Hawaiian issue. They were in fact declaring him — and his vehicle — to be part of Hawaii, the sovereign nation, and answering to the traditional monarchical system that was, some might say, unfairly dismissed early last century.

When confronted by the cop, Ross responded, 'I'm sorry, I don't recognise you as my governing body. I am part of the Hawaiian sovereign nation and don't adhere to your laws.' How radical is that! The cop didn't know what to do, so he did the obvious — took him to jail where he could exercise a little authority and hopefully make some sense of this rebel. 'So off I went to jail,' recalled Ross. 'They lock you up for a while until they realise there is nothing they can do ... then they let you go. It's happened a bunch of times now.'

Ross showed me his 'Hawaiian Sovereign Nation' driver's licence and an interesting documentary on how Queen Liliuokalani — and the monarchical system of the time — were unfairly overthrown. The flimsy reasons for why the annexation happened were mostly found under the carpet. As is the case with many indigenous cultures, their flow was no match for the power of the 'New World'.

## HAOLES

The Polynesians first arrived by canoe at the Hawaiian Islands between 300 and 750 AD. Captain Cook arrived there in 1778 and was killed in a dispute one year later at Kealakekua Bay, near Kona. By this time, whaling was already an industry on the islands, with many ships docking in the waters. However, once the European and American nations saw the richness of the volcanic soil, the peaceful islands of Hawaii, once ruled by its kings and queens, began to get a taste of the outside world.

In 1893, with Queen Liliuokalani on the throne and the Americans already controlling a lot of its new industry, the United States formed a committee of safety, surrounded the queen's palace with troops and declared the monarchy over. With American troops on her doorstep, Queen Liliuokalani was forced to surrender, and in 1894 the Republic of Hawaii was established. Later, on 12 August 1898, the government of the republic transferred sovereignty to the United States. Hawaii, through no choice of her own, became a territory of the United States in 1900. And although the queen received promises that there would be an immediate and fair investigation into the annexation, it never happened.

Eventually, even the American President Grover Cleveland declared that the annexation had been unlawful. He admitted, 'By an act of war, committed with the participation of a diplomatic representative of the United States and without authority of Congress, the Government of a feeble but friendly and confiding people has been overthrown. A substantial wrong has thus been done which a due regard for our national character as well as the rights of the injured people requires we should endeavour to repair ...'

'There are all these lawsuits going down right now,' said Ross. He was so passionate in his own relaxed way about who he was, where he had come from and where he wanted to be. That was in 1997.

There has since been a war in the Middle East and as one of America's biggest naval bases, Pearl Harbor — which was bombed by the Japanese in 1941 — dominates the island, the majority of bumper stickers display the Stars and Stripes and the slogan 'These colours don't fade'. They aren't talking about the old Polynesian flag, the extinct trees, birds or language; they're talking about the American culture, the money it makes from the surfing industry, from the sugar and pineapple fields, and from the high-rise hotels that accommodate the Japanese tourists who come to Waikiki every year. The big ancient head sees it all and yet he knows the spirit of aloha will never fade, because it is in all things natural: the volcanoes, the pulse of the waves and the hearts of everyone — even the *haoles* or tourists.

## THE SULLIVAN SHOW

His skin might not be quite as dark as the Polynesians', but his frame, built with muscle and peace — and the salt flowing through his veins —

makes Pancho Sullivan (number seven on surfing's World Championship Tour (WCT) in 2007) one of the most respected Hawaiians.

There is an ancient wisdom in Pancho; there isn't much he hasn't seen or experienced in the last thirty-four years of life on the North Shore.

'It's probably bizarre for some people, but it's a common story in Hawaii. I was born into a hippy commune on the Big Island, moved to Oahu when I was four and grew up on the North Shore. I was just the full surf rat, bouncing around from house to house. I grew up with my mom. She was a single mother and always working so I kinda had the freedom to come and go as I pleased. Because of that, I grew up without parental supervision, so the ocean became my protector; it's where I got my love and joy and contentment. I never had siblings, but I had a lot of friends I'd consider family. It's still a small town but back then it was even smaller and we just did whatever — just running amok, causing havoc, picking fights; whatever we could think of to keep ourselves occupied.'

Highs and lows are married in the Hawaiian psyche. Massive waves come, inspiring the adrenalin-charged instincts of fight or flight and the one omnipresent reality they live with throughout the swell season — death.

'A death always sends shockwaves through the community, no matter whether it's someone you know or not, because it reminds you of how dangerous surfing can be. The elements that we are dealing with along this stretch of coast really make you think about being in the moment and looking out for each other. There's something that we have as surfers — that brotherhood — and the knowledge that we should always be there to help a fellow surfer in that situation,' Pancho explained.

'A lot of guys like Shawn Briley have proven in the past that it is 50 per cent or more mental than it is physical. If you're able to relax in critical situations, then you're able to survive and handle some pretty radical things,' he continued.

(Shawn was a professional surfer from Hawaii who simply charged big waves, building a reputation for fearlessness that bordered on stupidity. He wasn't fit, he wasn't even talented, but he would never pull back.)

Pancho first became famous for his tube, cutty combos at Backdoor and Off The Wall (OTW), but in recent years his surfing has progressed onto the world stage. He qualified for the 2006 World Championship Tour and finished in the top ten in his second year of competition. He has evolved greatly as a surfer and is known throughout the world, but one place will always be associated with him.

'I've grown up all my life admiring people who can surf Sunset well because it's a tricky wave. It offers so many different aspects. You can potentially surf it like a small wave, so I've put in a lot of time out there — not so much for the contest results and reputation, but just for the pleasure of it.

'A lot of guys have realised that if you build a strong reputation out at Pipe and OTW, you can go a long way in surfing. It's such a tight take-off area and has such dangerous waves that you've really got to be aggressive and your ego has got to be strong just to be able to get waves. Sunset suits me a little more these days.'

Being ranked as one of the world's best surfers has been a long time coming for Pancho. First picked up by Billabong as an emerging teenage talent, then quickly scooped up by Rip Curl and heavily incorporated into the Search Program, Pancho travelled around the world making movies and taking photos. But his focus was always on Hawaii and surfing's Holy Grail: The Triple Crown (at Haleiwa, Sunset and Pipeline, during the North Shore winter). Always evolving as a person and a surfer, Pancho will have more trophies to come, but his wisdom and integrity are of greater value.

'I feel very blessed and fortunate to do what I do on a daily basis. I try to take complete advantage of that, and I surf whether it's a sloppy two foot or thirty foot. I'm pretty addicted to the ocean.'

## WATERMAN

Brian Keaulana once allowed himself to get cleaned up by an entire set at Jaws, just to make sure the jet ski driver he was teaching had the skills to be on the spot after each clean-up. He is universally respected as one of Hawaii's best lifeguards (in the true sense of the word) and has been an integral part of the waterman movement of the past three decades. When I caught up with him in Hawaii, it was at his 'Waterman's Day', a day when he shares the joys of water activities with everyone from the World Champion down to the local school kid. He lives on the West Side of Oahu; there are a lot of problems there with youth, so 'Uncle Brian' devised a plan. He set up heaps of stand-up paddle boards for the pros to ride. They brought donations. Surfers such as Mick Fanning and Pancho, who understand the problems, each brought three boards and a series of wetsuits and clothes. The idea is that they go into a loot. When a kid performs well at school, he or she receives credit points, which they can then use to purchase the booty. It is a great system and all the surfers had fun trying the stand-up paddle boards. Everyone from Mark Occhilupo to Mick Fanning was there to show their respect for Brian, the ocean and his heritage. I had a chance to speak with Brian during the day.

'I grew up in Makaha, on the West Side of Oahu. My father was one of the pioneer surfers, kind of a legend in his time. One of the first surfing competitions in the whole world was the Makaha International. I watched guys like Greg Noll, Buzzy Trent and Mickey Dora; then Gerry Lopez, Dane Keloha and Mark Richards. It's been a great life for me.

'My background is not only as a professional surfer, but as an ocean lifeguard in Hawaii, so basically I'm a waterman. I can do all sorts of water sports: wind surfing, kite surfing, canoe surfing, body surfing, bodyboarding, stand-up paddle surfing — any type of water sport. To us, a waterman is someone whose lifeblood is the water, someone who just purely enjoys the ocean. The ocean is a place where they can release all their stress and find serenity and calm and release. It is also basically a training ground in survival. It will console you and feed you.'

In his role as a lifeguard, Brian has seen and experienced some heavy situations.

'Some of the gnarliest things happen when you have an increasing swell that comes up from zero foot to twenty foot within an hour. All of a sudden guys are in way over their heads. They get afraid to paddle in and they're trapped, way out at sea. Rescuing those people is always heavy. Statistically, nearly all accidents happen in three foot of surf or under. You really just have to know your abilities and limitations. When we talk about respect, or surfers who respect the ocean, we mean the kind of surfer who will go out and study the spot. They'll ask questions. That's giving respect to the place, and that makes it far less dangerous.

'I try to train myself in the essences of strength, agility, flexibility and endurance. That's the acronym for safety. It's like the fingers on your hand. You can survive with probably four fingers, or even three, but having five fingers means you can do many more things. What a lot of surfers don't understand is that energy is oxygen when you're fighting the surf under water. You have to know when to use that energy and when to relax. You can't fight the power of the ocean. You have to know when to conserve the energy, and when to kick to the surface.'

## THE GOLDEN TICKET

During the main round of the Op Pro at Haleiwa, season 2006, I walked along the beach to go for a swim in between heats. It was a typical day in Hawaii; thick bands of clouds came in from the volcanic mountains, providing refuge from the burning sun. Sometimes they bring rain, and with it the most beautiful rainbows.

I bumped into Fred Patacchia senior, father of World Tour surfer Fred Patacchia junior. I said hello and together we watched his son surf his first heat in the Op Pro. The waves were four to six foot — and the ripbowl that is Haleiwa was proving itself to be one of the world's best high-performance waves. Binoculars in hand, Fred senior felt just as proud watching Fred junior as when he, Fred senior, was just a little world-beater, taking down people at this same beach.

Fred senior, a Californian, married a local Polynesian Hawaiian and moved to Hawaii in the seventies. He really appreciated his new life, and together with his son, put plans in motion to repay whatever Karmic energy had blessed them with their life in the Aloha State as professional surfers.

'He has his movie premiere on Saturday night,' said Fred senior about his son's new film. 'And all proceeds go towards local surfers. Fred got his start at this local Hawaiian level, you know, and he just wants to pass that on. Every year he has what he calls the "Golden ticket". He pays for a return ticket for highest placed junior who makes the NSSA finals and is without sponsorship, for them to compete in California and have their chance. Last year the guy came second — and Fred paid for his mum to go as well.'

'Yeah, it's something I'm so stoked to be involved with, you know?' said Fred junior.

Fred senior added, 'Hawaii is the home of surfing and there isn't too much help for the kids coming through. Surfing has given Fred so much and he wants all these kids to have the same chance that he had.'

## HAWAII

Hawaiian surfers have consistently been at the forefront of surfing since The Duke first introduced it to the modern world early last century. Hawaii has the best waves and the best blood. From Dane Keloha to Sunny Garcia, from the Irons brothers to the Hos, riding big waves is in their blood and in their backyard. If a title was awarded for the number of champion surfers per capita, no country would even come close to the state of Hawaii. And that admission is coming from the proudest of Australians. A surfer here is a part of something very special, an honour passed down by their elders. It's not just the 'Aloha State', as the licence plate suggests; it's an aloha state of being that connects Hawaiians to the ocean in a more powerful way than any other people except one — the Polynesians from whom they came.

## ICE MAN

There's a certain relationship with adrenalin that every surfer from Hawaii shares. From an early age, for seven continuous months of the year (October to May), Hawaiians surf big waves — really big waves. The sound of the ocean exploding as rhythmically as the ticking of a

[10]  a wave away

clock keeps them awake at night. Swells get so big that you ring your family the night before. Your breathing changes with a new appreciation of oxygen. Fear and excitement flirt with life and death. And then, in June, it all stops. The ocean goes flat and the adrenalin with it. It is for this reason that a lot of people have turned to drugs as a substitute for the feeling that surfing big waves inspires.

These days trouble comes in an ice pipe on the North Shore. 'Ice has caused so many problems here. There might have been a joint being passed around when I was growing up; now it's an ice pipe. It makes people really aggressive; they steal. And because it's so cheap and accessible, so many kids are having it put in front of them. It's a very serious problem,' explained Pancho.

Cocaine, speed, marijuana — it's all there. But when ice came to town, things changed. Then of course there's the money involved with drugs and the North Shore hierarchy soon muscled in to take charge of the drug cartel — paying off police, strong-arming local dealers. Between the waves and the volcanoes, there's plenty of smoke clouding the aloha spirit — but most of it comes from drugs.

I was in hospital one day a season ago, getting a cut stitched up. Fathers, cousins, friends, kids — they were all coming into the hospital yelling and screaming, pushing and shoving. They were off on ice.

## THE LOCAL

'What do you think Log Cabins would be like today?' I asked Nolan. We were sitting at Sunset, checking the surf, and a strong north swell lined through Sunset Point. It was peaking up periodically at Sunset, but it was not quite big enough. Nolan looks like any other generously proportioned local. He's a big boy, at least 115 kilos: relaxed and full of aloha spirit; big and jovial. He grew up on the North Shore and has surfed there all his life. However, age, family and girth are now slowing him down. He turned around to show me the back of his head. Even the thick black Polynesian hair couldn't hide the scar that told the story of a hideous wipeout that almost killed him. 'My leash wrapped around the rocks on a big wave, bra. It stopped me in my tracks and whipped me back onto the rocks head first. That wave is dangerous, bra.'

Nolan now lives on the East Side, but has roots everywhere. 'I have ten brothers and sisters, bra, and they all have kids that are surfing now, so I'm pretty much related to everyone on the North Shore.'

Anyone who appears Polynesian on the North Shore is family. But there is one whose features seem to be chiselled from the volcanic rock itself. His long Polynesian hair flows like a palm tree in the wind and his spirit is as fresh and ancient as a wave.

Titus Kinimaka is a professional surfer, stuntman and adventurer, the new and evolving example of how much the sport of kings has developed in Hawaii. Titus lives on Kauai, and has discovered a way to earn a healthy living (physically, spiritually and economically) in the ocean. In 2005, at age fifty-one, Titus placed eighth in the Eddie Aikau Memorial event at Waimea Bay and, while he is still a sponsored surfer, now spends most of his time with the Hawaiian School of Surfing, a school he built into one of the most productive schools in the islands. I chatted with Titus a few years ago. Only days before, his fellow islander, Bruce Irons, had won the event. Titus speaks with the aloha spirit and remains true to his roots.

'Kauai is a little more laid back than here on the North Shore,' he said. 'For me it's really important to carry the spirit of surfing and to pass it down. We have some really good surfers on Kauai. The Irons brothers just blow me away. I've been watching them since they were kids and I'm so proud to see them do so well.'

## JAWS

The island of Maui is a place in itself. Like Kauai, it's a little remote and untapped by the hordes of surfers that come to the islands every year. It's green, full of volcanic mountains and misty waterfalls and surrounded by majestic blue water. But some of its waters have teeth!

'Jaws starts breaking at around ten to twelve feet,' said Ian Walsh, who is part of the new brigade of tow-in chargers. This guy is as ballsy as anyone, and he has already collected a mountain of stories in the pursuit of his madness. We were driving around the bay at Waimea with Mick Fanning, talking about big waves and about Jaws — the Mecca of them all. A huge swell was approaching and a friend of ours had organised a ski for us. I was hoping I would be mostly driving, but so was Mick.

'Put it this way, when Waimea is big, then Jaws will be almost double,' Walshy explained. Mick and I looked at each other and I could feel my intestines curl up in fear. We asked him more about Jaws to fill the silence.

'In the last big swell I almost drowned,' he said. 'I mistimed my run-in and had to take the drop again. So I kinda took a bit of air under my board as I free fell. I was really deep and I tried to bottom turn up into the pit, but just got mashed. The wipeout tore both my life vests off and they choked me. About a minute later I blacked out for a little while. I was down for so long and wasn't coming up, so I opened my eyes to see which way was up, you know, but there was no light at all. It was pitch black. A wave went past and then I came up in front of the next one, a thirty-foot whitewater which I wore on my head. Apparently my driver came past, but didn't have time to pick me up. He said I gave him the thumbs-up and told him I was cool. I don't remember any of that. I was half unconscious.'

## UNCLE RABBIT

His name is Rabbit Kekai, but people just call him Uncle Rabbit. At eighty-five years old, Uncle Rabbit is a living legend; he was baptised in the early days of the Waikiki Club, and mentored by the great waterman Duke Kahanamoku himself. He is armed with dirty, cheeky jokes and as much aloha spirit as the ocean itself. I sat with him during the Pipeline Masters in 2006, and we spoke of almost a century of aloha.

'I started surfing when I was four or five years old,' said Rabbit. 'That was in the twenties and we had the big redwood balsa boards. Duke taught me how to surf. There was a competition one day, and all the older guys didn't want me in it catching waves, but Duke told them to let me catch waves. He said, "Let the kid go. He's with me." From then on, I was in the club.'

The Waikiki Club was formed in 1905 by a nineteen-year-old Duke. He called it Hui Nalu, 'The Club of the Waves,' and it was where modern surfing was born and from where it spread. As their skills progressed, the club's members ventured from the easy waves of town to the outer reefs, pioneering some of today's most famous — and some still underground — big wave spots.

'We used to surf this spot called Bluebirds. It broke so far out to sea off Diamond Head, where only the birds would go. We would have to get a boat out there or spend most of the day paddling. Plus, we never had leashes in those days, so whenever you fell off, you had to swim in.' Rabbit laughs, knowing that the pain of all that effort is now behind him. 'One day a boat came through the line-up, on the inside of the break. A big set came and ...' Rabbit chuckles, remembering how massive that wave was. 'The guy in the boat must not ever have seen a wave break here before, because it only breaks every few years — and it was big.

'We started surfing Waimea in the thirties. Greg Noll and Fred Van Dyke say they were the first to surf it in the fifties. You know what I say to that?' He held his hand up high and raised his middle finger. 'I say to them, well, Dick went down in 1943 [in 1943, Woody Brown and Dickie Cross got caught out in rising surf at sunset and tried to paddle in at Waimea; Cross was never seen again], and we had been surfing it for a decade before then. If he went down in '43,' he said this nonchalantly, almost like a war veteran, as though death is part and parcel of surfing the waves, 'then how could you be the first more than fifteen years later?' He once again raised his middle finger. 'The day Dick went down was big. I mean, closing out from backyards across all the outside reefs. We are talking about a fifty to sixty foot swell here; something many Hawaiians haven't seen in their lifetime.'

You've got to take your hat off to those pioneers of the bay, especially Greg Noll, Mickey Munoz, Mike Stange, Harry Church and the few others who paddled out on their forty-pound planks and gave birth to a new cult in 1957.

Rabbit continued his stories.

'A little after we began surfing the bay, the Japs came and bombed Pearl Harbor. Things got weird for a little while then. We couldn't even surf the Pipeline because there was barbed wire all over the beach. They didn't know if there would be another bomb and Hawaii had become a war zone.'

The semi-finals were about to go out and Kelly Slater had just collected his competition rash vest from Uncle Rabbit. Rabbit is the one element that has always been here, even way before Kelly's time. Since the start of the competition, Rabbit has not missed an event in Hawaii. He is like family to all these people. He threw in a new dirty joke for the man he'd been giving contest singlets to for over fifteen years. 'Thanks, Rabbit,' grinned Slater and off he went to surf his semi. It was the year he won his eighth World Title. Many of them had been won at this very break — and every one of them had been witnessed by Uncle Rabbit.

'How has Pipe changed?' I asked.

'Pipe was more of a peak back then. There wasn't as much sand.'

'And surfers? You've seen everyone from the Duke to Kelly Slater. Who rode these waves the best? Or when was the best era?' Beneath the questions I was trying to tap into that wisdom myself, to try and get a feel for who he is, what surfing is to him, what Hawaii is to surfing. I was attempting to paddle to the horizon, but he brought me back to the simple realisation that dawns on every surfer when they first attempt to ride a board.

'There has been no better time, or no better surfer,' he stated. 'The ocean changes, the times change … and we gotta change with it.'

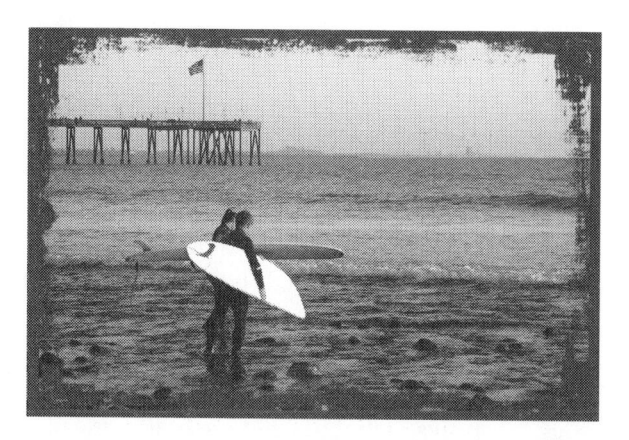

# STARS AND STRIFE
## USA

'These colours don't fade.' As in Hawaii, the sticker read loud and proud from the back of a Chevy truck as it made its way down the 405 towards San Diego. It was a typical weatherless day in California: dry, no clouds, little wind and a slight haze robbing the sky of its true colour. I regarded the sticker from the car behind. It boasted America's insignia of strength beneath the words — the stars and stripes — but the car was covered in rust. Defiant, the sticker remained fixed in a symbolic gesture, unifying strength above decay. I wondered if the owner even knew about the corrosion. He had just driven past Trestles, one of America's most famous surf breaks. To his right, a nuclear power station was between him and the beach. To his left, an explosion indicated that war games were being conducted in the hills where one of America's biggest army bases is located. He was surrounded by the stars and stripes of America, driving a massive car fuelled by petrol subsidised by tax cuts, erupting carbon dioxide above the twelve-lane freeway built by a corrupt government waging war on an idea.

What is — or what was — the idea of America? We could say it started with a bunch of disparate and opportunistic people, who, with little in common but the desire to choose their own paths to wealth or heaven, rallied behind the Declaration of Independence to build the richest, most inventive and most powerful country on earth. But with everything that's been going on in recent times, what does it actually mean to be American now? I pondered this thought as we followed the car down the highway.

## FORT KNOX

Taylor Knox is a man of exceptional range. As a surfer, he oozes integrity, displacing water with a unique combination of power and precision. In an understatement, he surfs the right way. He lives his life the same way, adhering to the natural laws of balance and flow. He just seems to do everything right. One minute he's debating environmental issues, complete with spiritual insights; the next minute he's making jokes and acting like a carefree child.

He is often referred to as 'Captain America' and I've always wondered why as I have never seen him as passionately patriotic. But as I've come to know him better I've realised it's because he is the ideal person that everyone else wants to be like, surf like and live like. Nobody is perfect, but this guy attempts it on a daily basis.

A good place to begin to understand American surf culture is through Taylor's eyes. He is also a writer and he preferred to write his answers to my questions. I quizzed him during the Hawaiian winter of 2007, in between surfs, training sessions and just everyday living. His first excerpt was scribed one morning in late November. He had just lost in the quarters at Haleiwa the day before and we were a little hungover from the previous night. The coffee was fresh, trade winds blew the palm trees gently outside our room at Sunset Beach and the surf was small.

'What was it like growing up in the action sports capital of the world?'

'Southern California is an interesting place in which to grow up. Yes, there are plastic people around and pockets of extreme materialism. These are facts, which have made some people a little negative. But I still have dreams about being able to change with the times. I live in such a great and inspiring place [North San Diego] as far as people in X-sports are concerned. I don't know why but everyone involved in these sports has ended up here and they make up a good percentage of the population. So when I go down to the Pannikan for some coffee and see Danny Way it's no big deal; we sit down and talk about the school that our kids go to and experience just sitting down like everyone else. But then we can talk on an athletic level and it's a pretty cool thing when you consider what he's done on a skateboard. It's nice to have that mutual respect for where we both are in our fields, but also to motivate each other.

'It's also cool to paddle out with these guys and see how much they love catching waves, and then have them invite my son and me to watch Bob Burnquist go and do the mega ramp at his house which is only ten minutes down the street. It makes me feel like a little inspired kid. It seems like I'm moving in that direction every day and this area gives me so many opportunities.

'It's amazing to have so many great athletes in the same area. I mean when you think about how many X Games gold medals there are within a ten-mile radius it really blows your mind. Whenever I feel a little uninspired I can just go down to Bob's house and watch him or Tony Hawk do the mega ramp. Wow! I don't walk away from that. I run to my car and jump in the water to sharpen my surfing tools and push myself to look at turns and airs differently. Sometimes you'll catch a few extra waves because you remember those guys throwing themselves off the ramp one more time even when they were exhausted. Not to mention how those guys are using their publicity for some great environmental awareness. In fact they have inspired me to convert my diesel truck into running on veggie oil. Everyone is starting to go in that direction, making more and more environmental products.'

It was early December. Knoxy had just lost at huge Sunset, only needing a 3.5. He had trained hard for it and deserved a big result. Sunset can easily humble aspirations with one misplaced set, and although he knew this one was beyond his control, he still took it pretty bad. We were back at the house, brown rice was boiling, and fresh *poky* — a Hawaiian tuna dish — and a spinach salad were waiting to join us for dinner.

'How would you say the American surf culture differs from the surf culture in the rest of the world?'

'Well it was interesting growing up in two different areas that view competition in a different light. I learned to surf in Oxnard, which at the time was really against contest surfing. When you're young it doesn't matter because it's all about the love of being in the water. Those guys were all about black wetsuits and white boards with no stickers and being humble. Well, in part that is. They really defended their breaks — and sometimes that meant with aggression. So I guess that's not exactly humble, but it was part of the heritage that came with that area.

'In fact, when surfing in California really started to explode in the fifties with Mickey Dora at Malibu it had nothing to do with contests at all. It was all about style. If you wanted respect from your peers and magazines, it was all about your style in and out of the water. That's where Oz was different to us. They were into the contest thing and it wasn't looked down on at all.

'I read every magazine I could get my hands on, which kept me in the loop of what was happening out in the world. And it was Tom Curren who inspired me to want to compete. He didn't lose his great fluid style when he put the jersey on and was humble when he was on the podium. I don't know if I would've been able to continue if I didn't move to Carlsbad in eighth grade. It was like moving to a different country. There were so many great surfers. The contest thing was widely accepted and the NSSA (National Series of Surf Associations) was in full tilt and I jumped in head first.'

Taylor won many events and quickly began his rise to stardom with style and humility. What made it even more special was who he was competing against and beating.

I stirred the rice and changed the music.

'You were part of the Momentum generation [a generation of surfers who produced big-hit surf movies under the direction of Taylor Steele], one of the most influential of our times. What influence did that have on you and what do you think you brought to that group?'

'Big question. Looking back on it now I feel so lucky to have grown up in that group. You have no idea. You've got to remember that there have always been certain groups coming up through the ranks all the time, but for a group to be that big was unusual. The fact that Kelly was leading the charge was a huge point. Watching someone with that much drive and determination not becoming sidetracked with drugs and fame was unique. We became so competitive in the water and on land it was like you had to be on all the time; you knew the other guys were watching so when you did something good it put a little spring in your step. And when you were bogging you would get down and dig deeper for the next session. After a couple of years people started pulling apart as far as their styles went. I went into the power side of surfing, wanting to have the best carving turn.

'It's interesting talking about being "on" now at this point in my life because of the introspection with my meditation. I mean, being "on" takes a lot of physical energy which at that time in your life you can expend on a seemingly never-ending source of adrenalin. I can see now how that was what actually held me back personally, because I didn't have a balance of knowing how to turn off. I only knew one speed and that was full throttle, and if you believe that the body follows the mind then it's easy to see how I could've given myself more time to trust my ability and not force things.'

An American sitcom called 'The Office' was playing on his TV. We laughed, changed the subject, put the computer away and ate our food.

A few days later we were preparing for Pipe, but the waves were small. The sand had built up and the outlook for the event wasn't good. Wade Tokoro — a surfboard shaper from Hawaii — had dropped some boards at Taylor's house, which joined the ten to twelve guns shaped by his long-time sponsor, Al Merricks. Knoxy didn't know it then, but none would be ridden. He ended up losing early in the Pipe Masters. It was two foot. He stayed for a few days to complete his program with our trainers.

We talked about the next year, and we finished the interview. The winds were still blowing from the northeast. They are trade winds and they force the palms deep into their stretch. The waves were still small and the event organisers were starting to panic. Knoxy made some coffee. Soon we would surf on our new bonzer bottoms. But for now, the computer came back out. He typed while I made a play list for our car.

'Why do you think you were tagged Captain America and what does that mean to you?'

'I don't know, I guess it started when a magazine did an article on the group and everyone needed to be a super hero. I always wanted to be Flash or Aquaman. Damn it! I always get thrown under the bus. Maybe it's because I look like the stereotypical all-American apple pie guy. I'm not sure how I feel about that. I guess it's better than being Wonder Woman or Batman's sidekick. It was never a patriotic thing with me. I understand it and it's fun to do team events but I know with the group [Momentum] it was never a country versus country thing.

'There's something different and very real about you in a situation where people are often vulnerable to becoming fake in order to move ahead or fit in socially. What do you think it was that shaped you as a person and a surfer?'

'Well, how far down the rabbit hole do you want to go! I don't think I went through anything different from a lot of other people: separated parents, divorce, careers and just normal everyday challenges. The thing that changed was getting to a point where someone could have looked at me from the outside and said "What the hell! This guy is not happy and he gets to do this for a job!" Basically I had to look somewhere inside myself that I didn't want to go to before. I was fortunate enough to meet an amazing teacher — and it wasn't some goofy New Age stuff. That was really a turning point for me — I started using my mind more than my brain.'

'What do you see for the future of America and for yourself?'

'America first of all needs to get Bush out of office and get someone in there who has serious concern for the environment. And as far as surfing goes, I think Dane [Reynolds] is the best prospect we have. There are so many juniors coming up that it would be hard to name all of them. Off the top of my head Brother [the son of former pro Dino Andino] and Duran Barr are two. But to me, what really sets a kid apart is if they are humble. The parents need to keep themselves in check though, because there is becoming an alarming amount of soccer moms and dads in this sport. And that makes a kid either surf for the right reasons or the wrong reasons.

'I still feel as if there's something untapped with my surfing. That's a big reason why I will be putting my best foot forward until I decide to change direction. And I don't see that happening for a while. I still haven't done my best surfing yet!'

'What is America to you?'

'A melting pot of cultures, which is really evident living in San Diego. I always wonder what it would be like if the world was one country. If travelling could be more seamless, maybe people wouldn't feel like they have to be so protective about their culture. The reason we have to have laws is because people can't seem to govern themselves. America gives me a big smile when I think about offshore winds, sage bush, swells like corduroy coming down one of our point breaks — and watching baseball with my friends after surfing all day.'

## THE LONG ROAD

I was in the car with Nathan Hedge (Hog) and our good friends the Long brothers, Rusty and Greg, in September 2006, and it was a typical day in southern California. The air was dry and the blue sky was losing its colour to a slight haze. It hung over the city and coast like passive smoke that even the rising sea breeze couldn't disperse.

The Boost Mobile Pro had been called off for the day and we were heading south of their home at Trestles and looking for waves. Rusty and Greg live surfing. Due to their command of massive waves, they have both won and placed in every XXL Award since its inception. You wouldn't pick it by looking at them. They aren't of Spartan build, don't talk like adrenalin junkies, or gargle nails for breakfast, but beneath their boardies are balls of steel. Hog and I stay with them every year that the Boost Mobile Pro is on at Trestles — and a better, more humble and aware family, you will not find.

Their dad Steve, a long-time lifeguard, runs the local state park (Doheny) and their mum is a primary school teacher over their back fence at San Clemente. They live in a peaceful little pocket of land in San Clemente. In fact, they are the peaceful little pocket in a high-rolling, fast moving surf scene.

On our way down the 405, Rusty explained an issue for Trestles' locals: a new highway that threatens the natural source of their wave.

'They are planning to put like 16,000 new homes inland from here. So they want to build a new highway right through the valley.' He pointed inland, over the dry hills that were scattered with brush. The valley looked beautiful; you could almost imagine the Native Americans hunting game there 300 years ago. But all around it is chaos. There is a nuclear power plant just a few kilometres down the 405. And just when I got that image through my head, I heard thunder slapping the silence. 'Oh, that's the army base,' said Greg. 'Blowing up something. They are right over there, over that hill. The base is massive and they are playing war games all the time. We grew up with those sounds.'

a wave away [25]

'It's one of the biggest army bases in the United States,' explained Rusty. 'It is seen as a critical and strategic part of the protection of this country. There are around 100,000 people on the base and it's an economy of its own, in around fifty square miles of land. It's in a really big zone of prime Southern Californian land. In a way it's good because it's stopped the urban sprawl from LA, but it's pretty bad in a moral sense. I grew up hearing explosions in the hills on a daily basis. We have massive noise pollution in that area: a twelve-lane freeway, the bombs in the hills, automatic machine-gun fire, helicopters overhead ... it's a really bizarre place to live. If you could beam the Native Americans into this place now they would think they were on a different planet.'

We drove past two massive hemispheres of concrete. They looked like huge breasts — and were surely built with a sense of humour. But whatever the view inspired in our own imagination, it didn't hide what's under there.

'The nuclear plant was built in the 1960s — a five-year project involving massive bulldozers right in the Mecca of surfing. A lot of American surfing history was built on that break — and now there's a nuclear power plant on it. It's pretty heavy. There were quite a lot of full-on protests against it back in the day and the old guys all talk about the day the bulldozers rocked up and destroyed their break.'

We turned off the highway and drove through the army barracks towards our surf. It's usually off limits, but Rusty flashed his card and curved his manner to the polite to gain entry. 'Hello, sir. I'm a lifeguard.' The car went silent as we waited to be let on to military ground. The soldier examined his credentials thoroughly as the American flag flew over his head. Seconds past like minutes; then we got the green light, and moved slowly through the barracks towards the ocean.

'There are around 40–50,000 soldiers living on this strip,' said Rusty. 'They have their own little economy going. Check it out.' Between the army barracks, munition depots, helicopter pads and training grounds, there are Burger Kings, petrol stations, lawyers, accountants, builders — all run by army personnel. It's not the environment Hog and I are used to. For these people it is their life. They live, eat, train, work and sleep on these barracks. The army — the defence of America — is their life.

We parked the car and walked over the sand towards the waves. An explosion startled me. Then a group of around ten or twelve army personnel ran by us, doing their morning training. They were dressed in camouflage with full training gear (yes, including guns), strapped to their bodies. Orders were given for a swifter pace just as they noticed us. 'Looks like we got ourselves a couple of surfy girls here,' said a black officer who towered somewhere over six foot five. I had no reply.

There are nuclear power plants on the beach, a neon capitalism you can't ignore, a war on terror that doesn't make sense — and plans for urban sprawl on land prone to fires and fault lines, where earthquakes and droughts threaten. The fact that the closest water source is over 200 miles away starkly outlines the fragility of the oasis they have built in the desert. I thought again about what Rusty meant by noise pollution — and wondered if their governator (Arnie) — feel free to laugh — could deliver some truth and environmental awareness to the spreading and defence of Tinsel Town.

The peaks packed some power and Dane Reynolds was also out there, two photographers flanking his every move. His aerial manoeuvres were matched by two fighter jets flying past. They travelled so quick they left the sound behind them.

We rode some fun waves, but with the nuclear power plant in sight, the sound of bombs going off and soldiers jogging on the beach, it didn't exactly inspire relaxed surf. At the end of the day we re-entered Rusty and Greg's refuge. If there is one thing America has, it's accessibility to everything. Whatever food you want, career, hobby, religion — it's all here in the land of opportunity. If you can't get what you're after, just go up the 405 a little longer and you'll find it. In between all this, Rusty and his family have found their own way, between the war games, the power plant on their beach, and the commercial progress of sprawling Southern California.

'I was fortunate to be brought up with an open-minded view of the world because my parents are knowledgeable,' said Rusty. 'Living on the edge of a state park, I had an upbringing most kids don't have. A lot of people are stuck in the commercial bubble, and that is what they become. I was really lucky.'

There are many fun waves in this area, from T-Street to Trestles, but in the winter months things can become a bit more challenging. Swells built in the Bering Strait track their way across the Pacific, hitting the Californian coast and creating some of the world's premier big wave locations, for which it is famous.

Rusty has been chasing the big wave thing for a while now. He spends his time riding, tracking or anticipating big swells. This passion has taken him to many spots, not only around the world, but also along his own coastline. He has organised his life so that if a swell hits the opposite end of the earth, he doesn't need to question what to do. It's go time.

'I first started surfing Todos when I was fifteen or sixteen years old,' said Rusty. 'Just kinda testing the waters at six to eight feet. We were really lucky to have a break like that only two hours away from where we lived in California. From there I guess it was just a natural progression.

'Eventually when I was seventeen, I got out there on my first proper day, got the biggest wave of my life, and the worst beating I ever felt. I went over backwards and handled it okay. I realised I could do this, and started hunting it full time. I've been able to hallmark some pretty special sessions around the world since.'

Rusty was lucky that his brother Greg shared the same life. Their parents taught them awareness and respect for everything around them and they take that everywhere they go in the world. They are now dominating most big wave Californian spots. And they do it by riding massive waves, not talking about it.

'It's a special thing to have a brother, a blood family member, who does the same thing. We can travel with each other and share experiences. We are relying on each other at a really vital level. If shit hits the fan, we know we can look out for each other, which is a very special thing. It makes us comfortable because you need to get to know the environment, shut off the nerves, hold your breath and relax and get some of the most thrilling waves of your life.'

The brothers not only put themselves on the map; they also highlighted their country in some extra large sessions in the big winter months in places around their own home. Together, they became famous all around the world when, along with Mike Parsons and Brad Gerlach, they first surfed Cortes Bank when it was at a massive size.

'I first learned about Cortes when I was quite young,' said Rusty. 'There are a lot of island and outer bommies in this area that really show great potential for big waves. I have some friends in the area that fish out there and they told us about it. Then we saw some solid aerial photos of Cortes Bank; you couldn't judge how big it was, but it was obviously massive. The guys from town, Rob Brown and Mike Parsons, had been on to it also. I went out there when I was nineteen, naming it one of the best big waves in the world. It's a hundred miles directly off our hometown. It's a pretty expansive line-up, the size of three to four football fields, with lots of waves coming through. With only the two teams out there, it was a chance to really surf big waves, to be precise and not get caught up with the hustle and bustle of the big tow sessions these days. With my dad out there watching over us, and my brother as my partner, it was a special day. We'd had a bit of tow experience before that, but that was it — it was in at the deep end.'

Rusty now spends all his time searching for the biggest, baddest waves around. And he is finding most of them off his own coast. But there are still some more discoveries for Rusty to make, another secret waiting to happen — and, as always, he's doing his homework.

'Basically, there's still another island in close striking distance that's rumoured to have one of the biggest waves in the world breaking on it. That's the next mission my brother and I have up our sleeve. We will have to sacrifice a day at another spot to do the re-con, but we'll never know until we go.'

## FEAR

Let's talk about fear, since we're on the subject. In some ways it can be seen as life's main opponent. It has truly domesticated us. Fear is a clever adversary that gathers momentum quickly, growing like weeds if left unchecked. It attacks your weakest point, always beginning in your head. It may express itself as self-doubt or anxiety;

then the mind clarifies the situation with reason — another clever ally in the fight against adventure. Fully equipped with reason, once fear takes over your head, it enters your body in the form of weakening muscles and shaking. Already your breathing has become shallow and your stomach contents have slithered away like a snake; your sphincter relaxed. You can postpone fear, but it will always give you the opportunity to face it. And it can be beaten, kept at bay, tinkered with. One weapon your body has is adrenalin. Adrenalin can quickly neutralise fear, giving flight to fight.

These days, extreme sports are taking over the action sports world — and one surfer leading the charge is Mike Parsons. 'Snipsy' has opened many doors in big wave surfing and lives the life of the old western cowboys but on a new front. He has prolonged his career and shown that while the human race tends to avoid personal contact with fear, people are very ready to relate to it from the comfort of their own couch. Thus a new boom has been born. And who better to make money from it than America?

Snipsy, like most, doesn't look like a charger. He used to be a top 16 surfer on the ASP World Tour. He never hit the lips hard or floated over big sections, but when the waves rose, so did something in him. Long retired from competition, Snips is now paid by Billabong, directing their events on the World Tour and liaising with anyone who tracks swells and learns how the ocean works. This guy lives life. If he's not chasing big waves around the world, he's hiking mountains and shooting rapids in canoes. Quite simply, Snips is not domesticated by fear. He is winning the battle and is an inspiration to everyone who isn't.

'It started with just me and Brad [Gerlach], over eight years ago now. We started doing it by ourselves without too much help. We got to a point where we had enough hours on skis and worked out a lot of things through trial and error. We are comfortable with what we're doing now.'

Like most things, it didn't just happen. His battle with fear was continuous and always evolving. Fear came up with clever tricks that Snipsy fought on every front.

'You just get in all these situations where, until they happen, you don't know how to react or what to do. A lot of times you're doing something wrong or you have to wipeout pretty bad to figure out how to do it. We're still learning and always changing our equipment. To become good at it, you have to put in a lot of time.'

His life has taken him to many dangerous places around the world, but he found the biggest and scariest of all close to home.

'The biggest waves I've surfed were at Cortes Bank for sure. The scariest wave I've ever surfed is Mavericks. It has all the elements — the rocks, the sharks, the cold. It's the eeriest place I've ever surfed. It just has that vibe. When you paddle out there, or even when you tow in there, you feel vulnerable. We're just trying not to make mistakes when it's really big. You're never completely confident. You're shit scared no matter what when a huge wave rolls you. I mean you can train all day every day but when you get nailed by one of those really big waves, you're totally at the mercy of the waves and vulnerable. So at that point, you're just like anyone else. I try to relax and stay calm, but really hoping for the best.

'My worst wipeout for sure was at Mavericks in '94. I took off on a wave behind Mark Foo [the late Hawaiian charger] when he drowned. Brock [Little] and I got wiped out and an entire set worked us. We got pushed into the rocks and my leash got stuck on the bottom. We were basically drowning. My leash broke and I got washed into the rocks, holding my board, and washed right over them. That was hands down the worst experience I've ever had in the ocean — ever.

'But the rewards are there as well. For me it is just being out there around those waves. It's not important to catch the biggest wave of the day. I just like being out there with my friends and testing my skills as a surfer. There's no better feeling than when you challenge yourself a little and when you get the ride of your life.'

This is where the trust in your partner and the camaraderie you share goes to new levels. Brad Gerlach explained, 'I need to know that he's committed to saving me if I'm in danger,' he said of Snips. 'So we trust each other in that department. Like right now, I feel like I'm bummed because I'm injured. When you think about it, we're a team and I feel like I'm letting him down. It's an interesting concept. A few days before Cortes, he was sick with the flu and I said, "Do you want me to bring you some soup? Are you taking your vitamin C? Dude, you better be taking your vitamin C!" It's funny, but all of a sudden you turn into this big brother. But it's good. He's a good guy, he's a classic guy, and he's got a lot of integrity. He's someone I want to be friends with for the rest of my life.'

## SANTA BARBARA BRUDDA

There are more than six million undocumented Mexicans living in America, over ten million documented. They wash dishes, cook food, clean cars, care for gardens. They do it for cash and they stay under the radar — of the government, anyway. But Mexicans are everywhere, especially in California. They are now a very large and important sector of the economy and culture.

One of them, in particular, has tattoos all over him, listens to hip-hop and wears a moustache. At first glance, some people would call him a gangster. His extra large T-shirt and shaved head would seem to prove it. But he's not. He's a professional surfer — the first Mexican-American surfer — living in a middle-income Mexican-American neighbourhood in Santa Barbara.

Because I think he's one of the coolest guys on tour — and because I have the pen — I want to write about Bobby Martinez and his place between LA and San Francisco.

Up in this part of California things are a little more green and pure. You can escape your problems and seek refuge in an uncrowded ocean that waves at you every day. The people are more down to earth and live relatively normal lives away from the entertainment industry of LA. This area has the Santa Ynez Mountains, Rincon, the Channel Islands and the wine country. And if that's not good enough, it also has Tom Curren, the 2006 ASP rookie of the year, who finished number five in the world in his first year on tour. 'It's a really good place to live,' Tom once told me.

Bobby Martinez likes it anyway — and he has the tattoo on his back to prove it. It says 'Santa Barbara Brudda.'

'There are so many point breaks up there, a whole series of them, so depending on the angle of the swell or wind, there is always somewhere good,' he explained.

The area suits Bobby, who doesn't get caught up in any of the bullshit of the surfing industry. It can be a little bit of a scene down in Southern California, where image can make up for lack of ability, where knowing someone can get you the gig, where standing out in the crowd by driving the biggest truck and having the best-looking girl is the way of keeping up with the Joneses.

Going for sponsorships that help sell clothes isn't part of Bobby's career. But he wins contests and has an incredible ability for riding waves. He keeps his skills pure, honest and hardworking. When it comes to results, he has both under and over-achieved. He won seven National NSSA titles, but then it took him five years to qualify for the World Tour. Then he won two events and became rookie of the year in his first year.

Bobby grew up in a place where the scene wasn't important, only who you had around you. During the Rip Curl Search WCT 'somewhere in Mexico' in July 2006, Bobby took some of his close friends along for the ride. They weren't even really surfers: just real mates from his real place. 'I'm lucky enough to be in a position to take these guys there and take care of their expenses. They are so much fun and have never even been on a plane before, so it's been a trip,' he explained. They watched him compete while the locals cheered for the guy they heard was Mexican — and they played soccer on the beach between heats.

We played with them when the event finished one afternoon. His friends were the same as him — big baggy shirts and shorts, tattoos underneath, shaved heads and moustaches over Mexican skin — but they were, like Bobby, just your average hardworking Mexican-Americans, born in America and living a life where your friends and family are the priority. For them, what you do for a living is an unimportant detail compared to the real meaning of life. They surfed, scored goals and smiled all day every day. Bobby lost in the event. But as hard as he tried, it wasn't the end of the world, because he comes from a place where other things have more value.

## MIAMI'S VICE

We were on our way to Miami for the premiere of Mick Fanning's movie, *Me, Myself and Eugene*. This is a loose part of the world where people know how to party and have a good time. Since all we did there was party and move on, I haven't got much more to tell. It was a wild night with wild opportunities on every front. Drugs come through there; so do hurricanes and space shuttles, models and immigrants. In one night we saw it all. Football and baseball are huge. Despite being the portal to the Caribbean and Latin America, the views and accents of the people are mostly rooted in the deep South.

'You boys call yourselves surfers? What is that anyhow? You ride boats or som'pin like dat?' 2003 World Champ CJ Hobgood and his brother Damien can mimic the accent perfectly, and it always makes me laugh. Though Miami has had its share of world champions — Kelly Slater, CJ, Margo Oberg, Lisa Anderson and Frieda Zamba — surfing is not a sport that registers high with the population of over seventeen million.

But that's not to say there aren't waves. There are waves; it's just that they're not very good. And the residents freely admit it. 'I learned pretty quick that to get waves, I had to travel,' said CJ. Though the peninsula has 663 beaches and 1800 miles of coastline, the waves are slowed by continental shelves and outer islands and there is a distance between the swells that build and disperse far from there. The Caribbean blocks south swells and the north swells are simply too far away. 'If it's breaking, there's waves,' he said. 'It might not break for three months at a time, so I learned to travel for my waves. I used to go to the Caribbean for three months every year. Then when I started doing contests it gave me more opportunities to travel and find the surf.'

'So it's that bad?' I asked.

'It isn't that bad. Yeah, well, maybe it's not so good.'

CJ and Damien Hobgood grew up at Satellite Beach, Florida. They have surfed through just about every NASA space launch — an achievement that is interesting all on its own.

'Because this is where the NASA launching pad is, there are hundreds of mad scientists around the place. It's an amazing thing to watch a space shuttle get boomed into space while you're surfing. There are all those people running around — and then there's a whole bunch of surfers. But where I live it doesn't even break for a few months a year. Sometimes when it breaks at home it's because of hurricanes. So just when we think there will be waves, we have to evacuate. It's pretty crazy. You see people driving over the bridge, evacuating the town — and then there are surfers driving in the opposite direction trying to get to the surf!'

Gabe Kling is from Jacksonville, the biggest city in Florida. It's further north from Satellite Beach and, like its people, somewhere between the vices of peninsula-minded Miami and the open-mindedness and opportunities of New York. 'It's pretty relaxed where I live. Not as touristy as down there,' he said. 'Everyone is into the NFL and they don't know very much about surfing. But if you want to party and hunt girls, down there is the place. So many models come from there it's a joke.'

In fact, there are so many beautiful women in Florida that a thousand new residents are attracted to move there every day. Hurricanes, floods, the heat and the lack of waves seem the only deterrent to Miami's vice.

## BEING KELLY SLATER

If somebody told you before 1990 that Mark Richards' record of four world titles would be beaten, you would have been coined an eccentric, an outcast with too much salt between the ears. Eighteen years later Kelly has won eight titles and become the first surfer to really earn mainstream respect. His surfing and his life is truly illustrious. It is for that he deserves mention. How he got there is one thing — but what's it like being Kelly Slater?

'Well I would say I was confronted with fame more than any other surfer in history. People sometimes call me by my acting name [Jimmy Slade] and when I won the world title there were headlines like, "Baywatch Kid Pulls It Off". People say it's an insult, because I'm not an actor. Ever since I can remember, surfing was the biggest thing in my life. To do the show really didn't take talent or anything. If they liked the way you look, you were in. I think it's radical that five or ten times more people know me for being in the show than from surfing. I have had people approach me not even knowing that I'm a surfer; they thought I just played a surfer. At twenty years old, I just wanted to be taken seriously.'

Fifteen years and eight world titles later, he is.

'Well it's funny because I have as much as I will ever need as far as money and material things are concerned. But I find the best time is when I have less things. I just end up surfing more. My life can be pretty complicated sometimes. As I move into this part of my career I'm really busy — there are lots of business and work opportunities. Then on top of that I have to keep my career moving with interviews, photo shoots and trips. And then I need time for my personal life — to keep in touch with my family and friends. I'm basically on the phone most of the time. My life's kinda cluttered, but when I need to I can always find time to be alone.'

These days, Kelly leads a fairly high-profile existence. In October 2007, for example, he went to Israel for a 'Surf for Peace' event. He was seen with Israel's top model and paparazzi chased him around all night, until finally he had enough.

'I couldn't believe it,' said Kelly. 'These guys were following me around all night and I was doing nothing. Then after about five hours or so I went back to the hotel with this girl and some other people. We just happened to both be staying there; it was no big deal at all. But the reporters made out like we were together. Anyway, I finally had enough and told the photographer to go home. He thought I was threatening him and said he had every right to be there. We had words and he called the police. He wanted to charge me with assault. He'd been following me around all night and I had done nothing! I rang up the guy who was looking after me and said, "Sorry, I know it's about 4 am, but I might need your help." I had to go to the police station. The police just told me to go home. But the next day I was in the papers all around the world for assaulting someone! It was so unfair!'

I guess all the fame escalated when Kelly first took his leave from competition (from 1999 to 2001), using that time to find himself and balance his life. But when he started dating Pamela Anderson, then Victoria's Secret model Gizelle, he became a little more famous and the balance was lost. Since then it's been hard for Kelly to find the flow back on tour, as he was no longer just a kid with high expectations; he was now the undisputed King with six world titles and a high-profile social life which he couldn't control.

'I think after having that time off it was hard to get back into a competitive frame of mind that felt healthy to me — one where I didn't get sucked into being too competitive in all aspects of my life. I didn't want it to consume me like that. I wanted to have a healthy, competitive approach where I was able to win or lose and still enjoy the moment.'

These days, Kelly is a bit of a vagabond, moving from place to place, still looking for that balance with life where things seem a little normal.

Right now, he is so accustomed to travelling that it is the only normal, or at least constant, thing in his life.

'You know what, I don't even know where I live. I've basically lived out of California for the last six to eight years. I spend an almost equal amount of time now in Australia, Hawaii and California, and some time in Florida. The rest of the time, I'm just on the road.

'During my early days on tour, I was actually engaged. It was more of a fantasy than a reality in my personal life. I don't think I realised that at the time, but with competition and travel, it was really hard to maintain relationships. I was getting home for really short periods of time. Most of my friends went to college and kept Florida as their base, whereas I had a whole new set of friends and a whole new life. I went from living in a small town to all of a sudden having everything thrown at my feet. I had all these opportunities to just do whatever I wanted. Luckily I wasn't into drugs [laughs]. That would have been scary. Overall, I stuck to myself a lot. And I would always get the cheapest hire car and spend the least amount of money — and I had the money to spend [laughs]. It got to the point where [his good friend and former world number two] Machado was starting to make fun of me. I didn't know any better. It seemed like the right thing to do because I grew up with no money.'

Things happened to Kelly quite quickly, and sometimes unexpectedly — like becoming a father.

'It scared the hell out of me. I was twenty-three, single, travelling around the world on tour and all of a sudden, I'm a father. At the time I really didn't feel as if I had my life figured out and I definitely didn't feel ready to settle down. I just had to become comfortable with it and let it become a natural part of my life. There was a part of me that was jumping for joy and another part of me that was terrified. All of a sudden there was something bigger than me and it was ready to grow up.'

Between travelling, surfing, fatherhood and Hollywood, Kelly began to connect even more to the ocean. The fact that he has won so many times in the last minute of heats would indicate that there is more than luck involved. Trevor Hendy (former Iron-man Champion and close friend of Kelly's) once told me Kelly had told him he could make waves come to him. It was worth asking him about.

'For sure. Everything in this universe moves in waves and patterns and when you can tap into what you are and how you do things in the purest way, I think you can transfer that to match the environment around you. I mean, I know that. So it's just connecting those dots and lines. When you're in tune with yourself you can easily be in tune with your environment and nature. My environment was surfing and the ocean and I've felt that. When you really tap into being happy and enjoying your life, then your full potential can come out. Most people aren't doing that — myself included. Most of us aren't really living from good happy places. But when someone who has a little bit of talent achieves that, they are able to do whatever they want.'

It is an interesting tangent. Kelly has also endured a real job.

'I've done all the acting stuff. I did some voiceovers for a cartoon and things like that. I think I had two different jobs that went for a day or two each. One was picking weeds. I got fired on the first day because I took too long. I thought I was doing a really thorough job.'

And what about retirement plans?

'I'll surf, play golf, travel. Being on tour is not something I want to be doing when I'm forty years old, but if I'm really enjoying it, then there's no need to make other plans. Unless I run out of goals or something. I'm not really thinking that far ahead yet.'

Though more world titles are not out of the question, Kelly's retirement is imminent. So the question remains: Can someone beat what he's done?

'Of course they can! I think it's going to take someone with real determination, but it can be done. If there's one thing I've learned, it's that whatever can be done, can be done better.'

## IS THIS PROGRESS?

Humans have a tendency to evolve. It happens without us even trying. It is one of nature's laws — we adapt; we learn to control and manipulate our environment to enhance our prosperity. We do it at the expense of others. And sometimes we do it at the expense of our environment. As the world's strongest economy, America — along with its allies McDonald's, Burger King, Wal-Mart and Starbucks — is leading the charge to world domination and destruction. They govern shopping malls in a forest of concrete, where expensive palm trees create an oasis-like illusion in what is, primarily, a desert. Like fake breasts, it looks good, attractively clean and alluring. You want to touch it, feel it. But it leaves you with a feeling of synthetic pleasure. It's a desert — and there's a colour and life that shouldn't exist. But it does — and this oasis is so well thought out and intelligently evolved that we believe it to be bona fide. But just as lips can be puffed and wrinkles can be tucked, so too can the landscape.

Just up the road from Knoxy's house in Carlsbad, millions of dollars are being spent on restoring the wetlands in the hope that the birds and fish will come back where the Native Americans and buffalo once roamed. The roads carve their way through the landscape, between the oasis cities, delivering their government-subsidised gas-guzzling trucks to and from the rich lands of economic opportunity. They're all coming to California. But what is the cost?

With 53 per cent of the country's population now living within fifty miles of the coast — and with an average of 3300 people moving to Southern California every day — there are certain pressures exerted on their coastline that the government is failing miserably to alleviate.

Below the neon canopy, all the run-off from the road plus 180 million gallons of poo takes the twelve-foot diameter pipeline out to the Pacific Ocean. It all comes to a dead end 4.5 miles out, waiting for the onshore wind to blow it back in. In nineteen storm drains along San Diego's best breaks, total coliform bacteria counts — which should be below 1000 parts per million (PPM) for safe swimming — are as high as 1.6 million. That's fancy talk for saying that between the nuclear power stations and the town run-off, the people are literally swimming in their own shit. But even more worrying is that this shit is no longer organic; by combining with the run-off from nuclear power plants and petrochemical engines, sunscreens and lip glosses, leaks from fake breasts and oil tankers, it's evolved into something very scary.

As more attention is paid to global warming, and high-profile athletes, politicians and movie stars bring awareness to it, maybe post-Bush America can swing the other way? Knoxy and his Carlsbad action sport buddies are converting their cars to run on vegetable oil. They have joined the Action Sports Environmental Coalition (ASEC). Could America, which led the world in industrialisation, consumerism and pollution, lead it back out?

The evolution of America has always been vulnerable to the one-sided aim of making money. But there are some realities they — and we — now face. You get the feeling that maybe the Americans who once rallied behind the Declaration of Independence in search of their fortune and conquered the Native Americans and drove them off their land — will shift their attention to what the Native Americans were actually doing when they arrived — respecting the land. So the cycle of life continues.

'Yes, I imagine it is the spiritual home of all things not real,' said Corey O'Malley, an Australian friend of mine whose vast intellect shuffles cards of creative eccentricity and clever design. 'What a shame that between New York and California, they have the world by the balls and can dictate what it wants to do and must be. Still, it could be worse. It could be, say, Beijing and Baluchistan driving the world agenda. Now I don't give a fuck what the bleeding heart hippies say from the comfort of their First-World left-wing expensive neighbourhood cradles; I'll take the crassness of American free enterprise and corporate killing over totalitarianism, facelessness and religious persecution by hysterical psychopaths in turbans, or Chinese "officials", any day. As long as their billion-dollar Yankee special cruise missiles don't slam into *my* investment properties!'

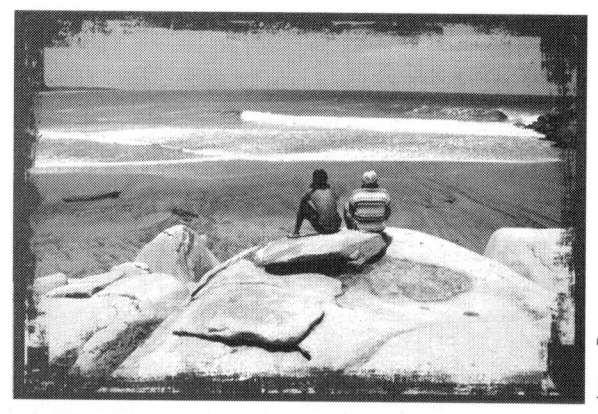

# SOUTH OF ... OPPORTUNITY
## MEXICO

'Check this out, it's unbelievable.' Mike Parsons had just sat down with Taylor Knox and me in a little bar at Mundaka, in the Basque country on the border of Spain and France. We ordered coffee — or a cup of 'fire' as Knoxy calls it — and prepared for the vision we were about to see. Mike set up his Mac computer on the table, found the QuickTime file that read 'Mexico' and hit play.

What we saw was vision from a water camera, taken as Mike powered up a river on his wave runner. The water was crystal clear, the river about fifty metres across. Frightened flamingos fled from his path, their bright colours hitting the blue sky in all directions like nature's firecrackers. Reeds lined the river banks and sand dunes made up the distance to the horizon.

'I have the camera strapped to a helmet,' said Mike. 'So it's cool. Wherever I look is what you are looking at.' This scene went on for two or three minutes and at no time was there any hint of human activity or influence, except for the noise of the 1200 horsepower Yamaha engine flying over the glassy water.

'Wait till you see this …'

He hit the ocean as the river broadened and became one with the Pacific. The water became broken and bumpy by the tidal pull of waves moving in multiple directions. There were sea birds chasing baitfish chasing bigger fish, but again, no sign of humans having ever been there before. He broke through the waves and out the back of the break. The water turned to glass again. Mike was with Timmy Reyes, World Tour surfer and a friend from California. He towed him into a wave — and we watched, through Mike's eyes, as Timmy carved in and out of the barrel for what seemed like kilometres.

'Oh my God!' said Knox. 'That was one of the best waves I have ever seen!'

'The best part is,' said Mike, 'that's just one part of the bank. It wasn't even the best part. We were moving up and down this point just chasing waves everywhere. And at any part of the point, waves were going forever.'

He clicked on another file and showed us more waves, more right-handers, more barrels, some birds — but no humans. The barman dropped a plate and Mike quickly looked over his shoulder, suddenly realising the fragility of his discovery — something he probably should be guarding like a mistress.

The word discovery deserves mention. It is a big part of the surfing lifestyle, and for no-one the saying 'It's the journey, not the destination' rings more true than for surfers. The satisfaction gained from learning the elements of nature, attaching them to geography, getting there — and at the right time — is and should always be the primary call for surfers with adventure in their blood. Just consider how many elements have come together, and the excitement of figuring them out. I'd never say where Mike's wave is; I didn't want to ask him. I just enjoyed the excitement of his journey, his spirit of adventure — and the result of his exploration.

Mike doesn't waste too much energy on such issues; he loves to share the spirit of surfing with anyone who carries it. Basically, he is the spirit of surfing.

'I drove down, took a week's worth of supplies, camped out at the riverbank, surfed and discovered perfect waves.' Mike had recently earned his pilot licence and does reconnaissance missions down to Mexico in between chasing big waves and directing WCT events, like this one at Mundaka. He goes looking for waves, often landing on the beach and surfing by himself.

At the end of that viewing, I knew two things: one, I needed to be better friends with Mike; and two, I needed to go back to Mexico.

When I first went, I was thirteen years old. My parents had taken me across the border during a family holiday in the US and it was quite confronting, even as a teenager, to be exposed to the social class system of Third World countries. But it does give you an insight into how lucky we are. We only went for a day, but I'll never forget seeing big Wal-Marts, McDonald's and Starbucks on one side of the border — people wearing expensive clothes and shoes, driving brand new cars like our hire car; then, on the other side, seeing people with old clothes, no shoes and no cars. It makes you question a few things. Thus was born my inquisitive nature from an early age.

Tijuana is the largest city in Baja California — that right arm that hangs off the body of Central America. That right arm that I'm sure US officials would at times like to amputate is one of the busiest borders — both officially and unofficially — in the world.

People are crossing to live on both sides of the borders; the Mexicans to enter the 'land of opportunity', and the Americans to lower their cost of living. The only difference is that the Mexicans are escaping and the Americans are mostly holidaying. Drugs, sex — it's all there. Moderate estimates say about 300,000 people a day cross the border into the United States — and who knows how many are crossing illegally? We do know that 11.5 to 12 million illegal immigrants have at some time crossed the border and are now living illegally in America. Drug and human trafficking is big business, crime is high and so is something else. Not too far away from all this, people come to feel the salt breeze of the Pacific. Some are getting more specific and finding that there are some of the best waves in the world in Tijuana.

The second time I went to Mexico was in 2006. It was for the Search WCT, 'Somewhere in Mexico'. I had decided to go early with my good mate Richard 'Dog' Marsh and surf Puerto for a week before the team came for the event. This is on the other side of Mexico where there are beautiful beaches and green mountains. Also, as this area is further south, it is more sub-tropical. The green mountains provide a beautiful backdrop against which to ponder the day's events over a Corona and a sunset. This is the postcard Mexico — where the waves are perfect; beautiful girls from around the world come with their backpacks and bikinis; there is little crime; and the beers are 50 cents and the tacos even cheaper. The south of Mexico points directly at the big south swells that come out of the deep Pacific.

'It gets huge here,' said Rusty Long, who spends a few months down here a year trying for the XXXL Biggest Barrel Award. He has bought property on the hill overlooking the left-hand point, and when he is not surfing you can catch him watching the waves from his balcony like a coiled spring, waiting for the biggest swells to start peaking. There are great restaurants here, great people and great waves. Since the onshore wind comes up around mid-morning every day, it's pretty easy to get into a smooth routine of surfing all morning, then relaxing in a hammock, reading a book and drinking Coronas all afternoon.

'Somewhere further down the coast is a series of perfect point breaks, some discovered, some undiscovered. You might notice a small aircraft flying over the top of some of them from time to time. Wave — because that could be Mike. If you were there in June 2006, you would have seen the best waves for a WCT event in history. 'That was actually quite lucky,' said Rusty, who came down for the week to hunt some other waves and watch the action. 'Only a decade ago, that point was pretty fat.' He pointed to the headland. 'The water was fairly deep over there, so the waves didn't really barrel and it wasn't a world-class wave by any means. Then they had a massive swell around ten years ago — and it pushed all this sand around the headland and created a beach.'

Rusty, his brother Greg, Dog and I were surfing it before everyone got there — and it was pumping. There was nobody around and the one or two people who did go out couldn't paddle against the sweep. Then another thing happened. Just before the event started, another huge swell came. To give you an idea of its size, it wiped out all the bars on the beach at Puerto, and gave Mark Healy the biggest barrel award when he got towed into a monster, forty-foot wave. At the point, the waves were at least ten to twelve feet. It was the biggest swell since the one that had brought in the sandbank ten years earlier, so more sand was being delivered to an area that was already way better than anything the world had ever seen.

I watched Mick get a seventeen-second barrel, then Andy and Kelly do it on the wave behind. Consider the luck: somewhere in the 4.6 billion years of the world's existence, after all the continental drifting, the rise and fall of water levels from various ice ages and meltdowns, and after the earthquakes that shook the land, the movement of the tectonic plates gave rise to the mountains and point on this headland that just happened to face perfectly southwest. A combination of giant swells in the last century broke and moved the sand into perfect position, until the last drops of sand arrived at the last minute. That last minute, in the scheme of things, fashioned the biggest low pressure system the Pacific had seen in decades, placed itself perfectly and maintained its form for long enough for the top forty-five surfers in the world to come here for the first time. I spoke to friends who have been back and it hasn't been the same since. Truly, nobody expected what they received. Such is the power and mystery of surfing.

The last time I went to Mexico was in 2007 for a training camp with the Rip Curl USA junior team. It was September, right before Trestles started. I had Kyle Ramey, Adam Wickwire, Alex and Koa Smith with me for four days. It wasn't far over the border, maybe an hour past Tijuana. As it's just over the border, it's obviously in Baja California — and we didn't have to go far to find good waves. We camped out at Enseneda — a place of expensive houses owned by Americans and rich Mexicans — and for four days we surfed our arses off, snacking on fish tacos in between. The land there is mostly desert; and being a desert, it doesn't get much weather, so we had to rely on long distance swells from the south Pacific. There isn't much local weather activity to confuse predictions, which makes it easy for long period forecasting. Whatever is on its way will get there eventually — even if it is a little tired. Waves have a pretty good reputation for eventually reaching their target.

A journalist from *Surfing* magazine came down for the day to shoot photos and write about the camp. He told us a story which, apparently, is becoming quite common in these parts. A police car flagged down two guys driving down the coast. They stopped, as you would. The police inspected the car, inspected them, and then did something peculiar. The police took the surfers' passports and they were told to wait while the police went to the station. The two guys didn't feel too good about this, but what could they do? Their bad feeling was unfortunately justified. Only minutes after the police left, the two surfers were robbed by the occupants of a new car that had arrived on the scene; all their cash, anything of value, was taken. When the police returned they seemed surprised. But anyone with experience of Mexico would tell you that they really weren't.

In Mexico, we surfed some fun waves. I trained some kids and showed them a few ways to improve before I had to get back up to California for the Trestles event. It was great being around their energy. On the way we drove past the island that is Todos Santos, one of the world's premier big wave spots. 'It's a scary wave,' said Taylor Knox, who won US$50,000 out there for what I still believe to be the gnarliest thing done in big wave surfing. It was around sixty feet — and he airdropped half the wave before re-centring at the bottom … somehow pulling it off. This was in winter when the water is colder, heavier and more dense.

'The thing about that is that only a minute before I got so pumped,' Taylor told me. 'I didn't make the wave before and got a two-wave hold down. I got licked, man. Then when I came up, I paddled for thirty seconds and that wave showed up. I was so pissed off I didn't make the other wave that I didn't even think about it; I just turned around and went. I didn't realise how big it was until I saw the photos. Mike Parsons is the gnarliest guy out there, though, for sure. Nobody comes close to him.'

As we drove past the island, I thought of Mike driving down for a thirty-foot surf. I thought of him launching his ski to take on the biggest waves out there; flying over the coast, over the border at Tijuana and into southern Mexico in a small airplane looking for waves. I remembered the footage of him camping at a river mouth, catching fish for dinner and driving his ski out to some of the most perfect waves you could ever see. Got to hang out with Mike more, I thought — and got to get back to Mexico.

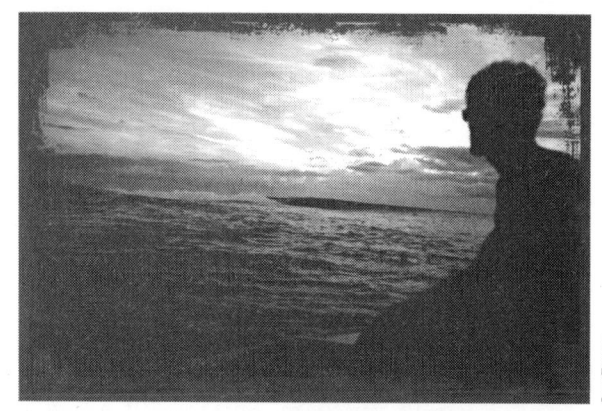

# KING TEAHUPOO'S GHOST
## TAHITI

With flowers placed around my neck upon arrival, I notice the soft caramel curves of femininity, the exotic cultural contrast of saronged-Polynesians bringing in local fish and washing it down with French wine, and the lush green canopy of soaring volcanoes climbing vertically above crystal blue water ... On a tropical volcanic island in the middle of the Pacific, you'd be forgiven for thinking that life is pretty easy. It can be, but below the surface is a unique oceanic spirit that defies words.

Take the road, for example. Like most things in Tahiti, it travels at the mountain's discretion. Basically, it goes where the volcanoes let it — around the tiny flat strip where the land meets the sea, where vertical mountains momentarily level to horizontal before sinking into the dark, fathomless blue. From the bay of Papeete, which is the hub of commerce and human activity, the road travels past the resident lagoon, with the massive volcanoes on the left and the active ocean to the right. On a big high tide and swell, or during a big rain, you will get your car's tyres wet. If both happen at once, then you start to get to realise who's running the show here. A few kilometres out to sea, the lagoon's tranquillity is lost to the turmoil of the outer reef, where small fish become big fish, ripples become big waves and crystal blue becomes an unknown dark. The reef has been formed by thousands of years of rain moulding the coral like a shaper would cut foam. Surfers will notice spitting barrels and small explosions, but you need a boat to get to them.

Clouds heavy with rain obscure the volcanic mountains and spill raindrops down the cliffs. Quite quickly, it finds valleys and forms rivers for kids to play in and for their mums to do their washing. The children play in the shore breaks on broken bits of four-by-two timber, left over from the house their dad built, and driftwood from landslides. Soon, they'll venture to the outside reef. There are houses along the road, and a couple of schools where the kids are taught how French is superior to the native tongue that only their grandmothers remember.

Soon, we are driving past Big Pass, a left that breaks as simply and powerfully as its namesake. It barrels and rides like a Hawaiian swell — and dishes up the same punishment when you fall. Further on, waves break in a scaled-down version at Small Pass. You might find surfers out at both these places, but generally not. Outside the reef, local fishermen chase big game like tuna and mahi. A single white bird will indicate that marlin are about and a bunch of black sea birds indicates baitfish — who in turn get eaten by mahi and tuna. If their hooks hold, thickset Tahitian mothers, fathers and their offspring will eat the tuna and mahi with lime and mayonnaise in a dish called Poisson Crue. Many fish dinners later, the girls will look like their mothers — big women with flowers in their hair, double pluggers on their feet and a sarong around their womanly bulk.

When you drive past their homes, Tahitians generally wave because the few cars that pass by are usually driven by another member of their extended, friendly family. Past the homes, and past the other secret reef passes, is a sleepy little village at the end of the road. This is a place where the mountains let you venture no further, so the road simply stops.

Up a little hill, a sign reads 'Teahupoo'.

Its name literally translates as 'hot head', and it marks a historical place where King Teahupoo's son once avenged the death of his father by eating the fresh brain of the murderer's only son.

Just after the Teahupoo sign, a church comes into view. It's a juxtaposition that makes you contemplate the afterlife and spiritual protection, even if prayer is like grasping at straws. Because of the wave's dangers, people have, will and should die out there.

While Tahiti's amazing atolls and reef passes have been a surf destination since the 1960s, it was not until 1982 that Teahupoo was first surfed by three local Tahitian brothers. As is typical when a wave is discovered, it was initially surfed quite conservatively, at its more playful and perfect size.

Thierry Vernaudon was one of the first guys to surf it consistently. He was out there in 1985 and soon started to push the limits above the playful zone. But it was in the late eighties that the infamous, backless walls, which seem to unload the full tide in one wave, were first attempted by Tahiti's favourite son, Vetea 'Poto' David. Poto had just returned from his second placing at the Pipeline Masters in the Hawaiian winter of '89 and, riding a big wave of confidence, took his much-publicised Hawaiian form and literally hitchhiked to the end of the road at Teahupoo.

'It was in May of 1990,' recalls Poto. 'And there was a big southwest swell. It was about eight to ten foot with a couple of ten to twelve footers coming through. It was just perfect. I thought I was at the Pipe Masters with nobody around. It used to take me three hours to hitchhike to Teahupoo, and as there were so many other perfect waves around my home, I didn't bother. But when I turned pro I bought a car and I started going there a lot more.'

Poto's lonely surfs wouldn't last. When the Gotcha Pro came in 1997, Teahupoo erupted, and the eventual winner Koby Abberton called it the heaviest wave in the world. Since then, the lava has continued to flow. The day before Mark Occhilupo won in 1999, he rang his wife to say, 'I love you — and there's a chance someone is going to die here.'

A year later, somebody did die. Local surfer Briece Taera attempted to duckdive a huge set, got caught on the reef and spent the next two days in a coma before dying. But that wasn't the end of the road as far as Teahupoo was concerned. In August 2000, Laird Hamilton rode through a cavern as big as the surrounding volcanoes. That wave was some kind of sick joke, and left the big wave veteran in tears. Since then, the most dangerous waves being ridden in the world have pretty much all been at Teahupoo.

The whole time, King Teahupoo's ghost has been been lurking, maiming and avenging. While the local community keep eating the fish, hula dancing and wrapping flowers around people's necks, more and more now attempt to surf the wave. A new breed of chargers have their fingers on the throttle despite the fact that, once it gets to a certain size — around eight to ten feet —

Teahupoo is only possible to surf with jet ski assistance. Yet the young surfers are ready for the rush, or perhaps the money and exposure that comes with it.

Nobody recognises the dangers as much as Poto. 'Everything you do there has to be calculated. You have to read the waves. If you don't have a sled and a life jacket, you shouldn't be out there. There is only a fifteen second gap between waves — so that only leaves three or four seconds to get in, get the surfer, and get out. I'm warning the whole world right now, for everyone that is coming in the future — if you don't have a sled and a jacket, I won't let it happen. I'll send you all in! It's too dangerous. It's becoming more of a business now and it's scaring me. People look at my shots and Laird's shots and think they can get deeper — and they probably could — but to the point where they kill themselves! This is serious business and people will die.'

Teahupoo may be the end of the road as far as big wave surfing goes, but where the road starts up again on the other side of the island, you'll find a different surfing culture. The crystal blue water that reflects colourful coral is replaced by black, sand-bottom beach breaks and points. Turtles roll up onto the beach to copulate, lay eggs, and continue the lifecycle; big fat locals drink Hinanos, play their ukuleles and laugh under swaying palm trees.

All are laughing except the men who are dressed as women. They are called 'mahoos'. It is a Tahitian tradition that every third son is born a female. They dress as a woman, go to the women's toilets, wear makeup. 'It's accepted here, but tourists always laugh,' said Alain Riou. Alain is one of the new crop of surfers coming through with Hira Terinatoofa, Manoa Drollet and Michel Bourez. 'It's so relaxed here; there are waves every day. The south side of the island works in the winter and in summer the north side gets all the swell. But there's always surf or something to do around or in the ocean. It's our life.'

Alain lives in Viroua, and just up the road from him lives his neighbour, Cote. Now a grandmother, she exudes a nurturing and mothering personality towards her friends, her family and the environment. One day, when I was eating avocadoes with her, she told me to make sure I planted the seed after I'd eaten the flesh. 'You must give back to the earth. Whatever you take from the mother earth, you give back — and she will always take care of you. We have food on trees everywhere. Lychees, bananas … you give and you take.' She also had some advice for surfing. 'Drink the whiskey before you surf and then you will dance on the waves.'

Further on are valleys which cut through the middle of the island amongst rivers and farmland growing Jurassic-sized crops, thanks to the nutrient rich soil from the surrounding volcanoes. The tide comes in and out. And just when you think you're starting to understand Tahiti, you learn that the tides never change there: it is low tide in the morning, high at lunch, and low again in the early evening. The time of the tide never changes. While I won't attempt to explain this phenomenon, I have accepted and subscribed to the solar reasoning. It was explained to me that the tides here aren't affected by the moon, but by the sun.

This made me think about the tides around the world. I don't understand tides at all, although, funnily enough, the Tahiti tide information seemed to make sense to me. After all, one would imagine that if the world's highs and lows balance each other, there must be a few places in the world where the water level is the same at all times. Backwash meeting forewash; high pressure water zones where all molecules agree to disagree. My question is — how does an ocean current deal with such an aquatic logjam?

Up at Cygnet Bay, in King Sound in northwest Australia, where a friend of mine worked on a pearl farm, the tides were wild. There was an eleven metre variation. 'It really made you think before throwing the dinghy anchor,' he said. We would power above large mangrove forests that, at low tide, were three kilometres from the water's edge. In places, the tide moved in and out across the immense flats literally at walking pace. And there was a three-hour time difference between the tides on one side of Cape Leveque from the other side — and they are only a twenty-minute walk apart. There were a number of horizontal ocean waterfalls twice daily, back and forth, as the water poured and roared over the ends of a few spits and reefs.

And another strange fact: Africa's Lake Malawi has bigger tides than the Mediterranean. The lake's tides are about five centimetres, whereas the Mediterranean's are only about a centimetre. I give up trying to understand the mysteries of the ocean tides.

In Tahiti you will sometimes find the occasional ex-pat Aussie, American or French indulger, living there and enjoying either the Tahitian lifestyle, or the beautiful ladies. The inland villages have supermarkets filled with baguettes, wine, cheese and anything French. They also have churches, thanks to early American missionaries. Some people believe in God, some don't, because there has always been something bigger rumbling in the Tahitian soul. Their acceptance of nature's extremes has led to their acceptance of other cultures. However, while their local religion and language may have been partially lost, the real culture will always remain. You can feel it beneath the green canopy of the red volcanoes, the thick rain cloud clothing the dry pinnacles and the crystal blue lagoons initiating dark explosions in waves like Teahupoo. It's nature at its most intense. You can see it on the drive around the island — the ocean to your right, the volcanoes to your left, and King Teahupoo's ghost sitting in the passenger seat for company.

TAHITI

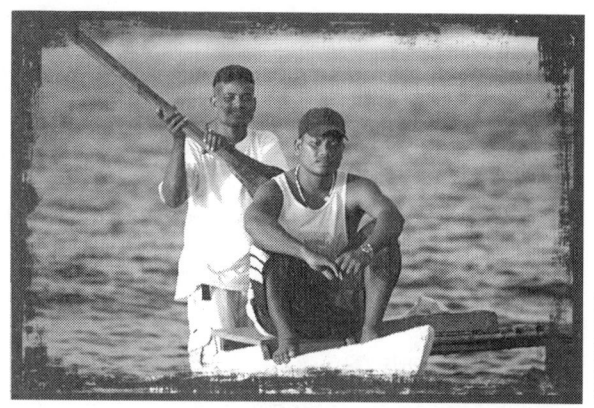

# THE NEW ARCHIPELAGO
## MICRONESIA

Monotones of soft greys and fluffy whites cloud the sky in these parts. They spill rain upon high mountaintops, Third World infrastructure and First World smiles. Simplicity floods, waves roll and the rain falls — constantly. Whalers used to come here, as did the wars of the world — hot and cold. As time passed, the winners wrote their history and their weapons sat on rented shores, pointing at paranoia. Soon, their weapons corroded, just like the power stations and fleeting foreign aid. And still the waves rolled and the rain fell. The Japanese fishermen came and went too, occasionally dropping anchor on the live coral. News of the amazing coral and sea life travelled back to Japan and tourists came to scuba under the fleeting sun and gawk at the colourful reef their countrymen were slowly destroying — until recent recession rusted the zipper on their wallets, and closed the booming hotels that had catered for them. Still the swells rolled in, the rain came and went, and the locals smiled.

Knowing nothing else, the locals continued to manoeuvre their dangerous reef passes in two-stroke powered canoes, trawling for tuna and marlin. They are good at it, despite the swells that test their skill and the Japanese that test their supply. Still, the rain falls and the waves roll. Despite years of human intervention in this massive archipelago in the Pacific, nobody had noticed that the waves surrounding this island were perhaps the best on this planet. Nobody had noticed, that is, until now.

After looking at nautical maps and swell charts for years, an opportunistic human (let's respect his privacy and call him Grommet) decided, like other foreign investors, that this island was worth something — though his investment was of a different and non-economic nature. He packed his raincoat, a couple of boards, some brown rice and came to an island that surfing had yet to discover. That was eight years ago and he is yet to leave, though he still ventures out sometimes for some brown rice to go with his fish.

Grommet wasn't the first foreigner to arrive on this island, but he was the first surfer. After employing local fishermen's boats for scouting missions on known reef passes, he found plenty of waves. Some were bad, some had promise — and none of them had been surfed before. He endured rain, lack of female company, strong trade winds, moody tides and was about ready to throw in his raincoat. Then he discovered his paradise — a pass where predominant swell directions and trade winds met face to face on a perfect reef set-up.

That was four years ago, some thirty years after surfers and hippies had mapped the holiday destinations across the world. 'You sacrifice a lot to live in a place like this,' said Grommet, who is more like the modern-day surf rat than the hippy of yesteryear — a brother from a different decade, though his blood is still the same. After his years of isolation Grommet is slowly, and very selectively, inviting others to surf with him in his paradise. 'There are not many girls, the food is terrible, but the surfing — it's unbelievable!' is his invitation.

Hawaiian Pancho Sullivan, another brother of the salty soul, had previously met Grommet and the two had corresponded for years. Then he earned an invite and brought a small crew of searchers for the journey. Grommet was toying with the idea of starting a low-profile surf camp in order to be able to keep surfing here and to give him someone to surf with. Thus the relationship was formed.

We got straight off the plane from across the globe — Kieren Perrow and Darren O'Rafferty from Australia and the rising WCT star, Raoni Monteiro, all the way from Brazil. Each of us had endured two full days of travelling, and we had no idea what to expect in this new place and new ocean. 'Looks like there is a bit of whitewater on the reef,' said Grommet, as if it were as constant as fish in the sea. Twenty minutes later, and about ten kilometres closer, that whitewater exploded in eight-foot bombs on a reef that looked the mirror image of Teahupoo. The rain fell, the ocean rose, and raw water closed in on this small island. Boards and legropes broke, blood was spilled and egos devastated.

The waves were about 100 metres long and, like Teahupoo, had two sections to it. The six-footers were perfect, but we would soon learn that the eight-footers, like Teahupoo, hit the reef with twice the ferocity. The swells climbed the draining reef, doubled up and tripped on the awaiting coral. Dangerous? Of course. But fuck — it was perfect! Kieren and Pancho were going mad, waiting for the biggest sets, but it was Raoni who got the biggest wave of the day. He stood deep in the throaty monster and put his hands to the roof, only to fall short by about four times his height. 'That was the best wave of my life!' he said, over and over. It was a four-hour session till dark. KP broke a board, and so did I. Pancho broke two fins and our skin was as burned as if we'd stuck our faces on a hot plate. But barrels were scored like never before.

'This is maybe the best wave I've ever surfed,' said Pancho. 'Nah, you know what? It is! I've never had so many barrels in one surf in my life. And look, there is nobody around.' He looked around and couldn't help but laugh. The mountains were lonely, the rain fell — and still the swells rolled in.

After the first surf, we were crying out for a bit of good grub. We knew there would be an abundance of fish and were looking forward to combining it with some fresh fruit and vegies. But there was nothing of the sort. A tropical terrain always conjures up notions of healthy living: papaya, mangoes and exotic fruits. But here there was no fruit — none! 'Apart from coconut and banana trees, they only grow things on the island that can get them high,' said Grommet. 'Betel nut and zakow, which they ferment into a toxic blend of alcoholic rum and slurp in generous mouthfuls out of sawn-off Coke bottles. If you try hard enough for a mixer, you can probably taste where the Coke used to be.'

It may have been just from the betel nut or zakow, but the locals also seemed to get high from watching the boys surfing. Except for those who were lucky enough to work with Grommet, none of them had ever seen anything like it before. 'Quick, run!' said the boat driver every time someone got in the barrel. He had been driving past this pass with his father — and now his son — for fifty years. He told us a story about fishing once with his father when he was only twelve, some fifty years ago. His dad was busy pulling in a massive marlin when his son fell out of the boat.

The father disregarded his son and kept fighting the fish for hours, while his son struggled to tread water in the turbulent ocean. He ended up marooned on the reef at low tide during the night, and as the tide came in, he had to swim back towards shore under the failing moonlight. He arrived back at his house around lunchtime the next day, exhausted. Luckily, his dad was there, cutting up the marlin for lunch.

Micronesia's location has made it strategic for expansive nations. The Japanese occupied the island during World War II and the Americans have been there since. While in Micronesia, the Japanese demonstrated their power with generators and cannons. And once the Japanese were defeated, the Americans started investing money in case they needed to set up their cannons in the future.

Old World War II tanks are rusting away on the island. And the new technologies that have arrived are also rusting away simply because nobody knows how to use them. Schoolteachers have been imported to teach the locals how to use condoms, grow crops, and to tell them not to eat betel nuts; dentists have been imported to pull out rotting red teeth caused by the betel nut; doctors are imported to cure STDs and to dislodge fishing hooks; and bankers are imported to take care of the imported money. It's all a bit too much for the local community, so they just keep drinking the zakow and eating the betel nut, more interested in the falling rain and rolling waves.

None of the locals surf. They are watermen, with diving and deep-sea fishing skills that would suggest, like the Hawaiians, a love of riding waves. But the notion has escaped them. This lack of a seemingly natural progression, however, has a reason. Unlike in Hawaii, there is nothing close to entry level surfing here. First, the passes are way out at sea and only noticed by the fishermen. Second, those swells rise out of the ocean in generous serves and, when the deep water suddenly becomes shallow, the waves seem to unload the whole tide in one motion. Who would think to attempt it? Better to chew the betel nut, negotiate the swells (not the breaking ones) and bring in the fish. The two or three lucky locals who got to watch Kieren, Raff, Pancho and Raoni were blown away. They knew the waves well and told stories of their venom, but surfing they had never seen.

'Imagine how many sec ... minutes we have all spent in the tube today,' said Raff. To even say that, you know you're having a good surf. But there was one day where video evidence showed the boys had clocked about ten minutes in the tube — in one day! I don't think we'll ever experience that again in our lifetime. Maybe if Kirra — on the Gold Coast — had nobody out you could get close, but this was something we'd never seen before. To be honest, there really is only one proper good wave here — but it is really good. This happened about three or four days out of the two weeks we spent there. I imagined how many days Grommet has had like that; how many intimate moments he has spent with his porno collection for company; how many rainy, flat days he has endured with the betel nut and zakow; how many more mossies and flies he has met than humans ...

Beneath the fluffy white clouds, rain spilled. So too did Grommet. He talked of all his hardships, his loneliness and his discipline. Then, from the raging blue, a wave rolled towards him. He swung and, to the cries of 'run' from the boat, engineered his way out of the barrel. He laughed as hardships became a forgotten memory. 'It only takes one wave like that and you forget anything bad that ever happened in your life,' he exclaimed.

I looked to the ocean as a set came. The water rose to my feet, the waves rolled and the rain fell. Eternal simplicity flooded beneath the clouds. The waves will never go away, but crowds could one day corrode this unique place. I just hope Grommet keeps his paradise for a bit longer — and that somewhere out there, the ocean continues to mystify and elude us in many more places yet.

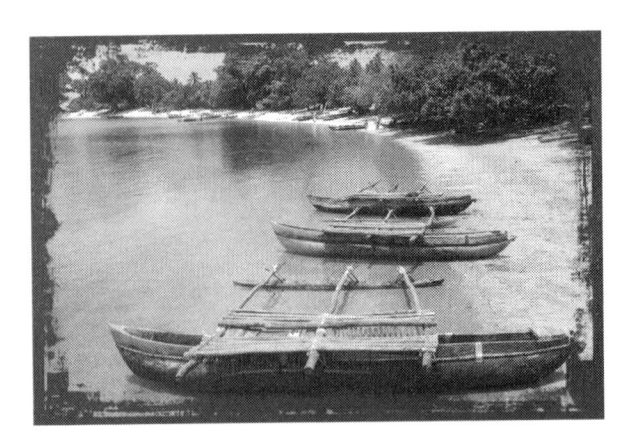

# WRETCHES IN PARADISE
## NEW CALEDONIA

To tell you the truth, I didn't even know where New Caledonia was. 'South Pacific.' That was what I told Luke Stedman, Koby Abberton, Clint Kimmins, Joel Bonning and Mark Mathews. They came along for the ride, also blindfolded to the possibilities and the geography of this mysterious island. 'It's French,' I knew that, 'and has some sick waves on outer reefs — apparently.' I coughed and lapsed into a mumble to cloud my uncertainty. I really didn't know much about this place and that humbled me. How could an entire island, especially one with waves, reside in the Pacific and I not know its dimensions and coordinates? The assignment got me thinking, that's for sure, and I was definitely excited about the island 'lost' in an ocean.

My research started in the office of Air Caledonie in the CBD of Sydney where I was waiting to pick up tickets. To get to their office, I had to elevate twelve floors, and walk past other airline companies. One in particular — Gulf Air — grabbed my attention. The world has changed a lot in the past few years. The lady behind the Gulf Air desk evoked images of religions and ethics so different from our own. She looked as if she hadn't seen a customer in a while and she sat like an ashamed little child, wondering what she'd done wrong. However, for all I knew she may have just finished doing her laps at Bondi Beach and was wearing the crumbs of her vegemite sandwich on her lap beneath the table. But — like most of us — I didn't get close enough to see. I smiled to let her know that whatever problems this world faced were not ours, but we didn't totally engage.

## ARRIVING

As I flew out of Australia, I studied the international map at the back of the inflight magazine. There she was. Sandwiched between Queensland and Fiji is New Caledonia. It's a large landmass, parallel to the Australian coast and so close it seems to be a part of it. It almost looks as if a chunk of Australia's Great Barrier Reef detached itself, floated away and turned itself into an island.

It was starting to take shape out of my airplane window — a lonely land awkwardly forming out of the dark blue. Its perimeter, the inside of the outer reef, sparkled turquoise. A series of small islands was dotted around, with empty sandy beaches running up into the dry mountains. It was the afternoon and the waves had already beaten us to the island. The wind gallops in there every day around 11 am, skimming across the water like rocks and pulling up as it reaches the fringe of the world's second-greatest barrier reef.

The view from the plane was amazing and I froze the short glimpse in my mind like a photograph. The dark blue of the Pacific flickered crystal where it became shallow to allow breaking waves to smother the coral. Inside the outer reefs, the lagoon turned a majestic light blue as we flew over it. Reef turned into shallow sand, then deep water again and scattered islands dotted the ten or eleven kilometres to shore. It was quickly obvious that you could not paddle out to the surf breaks, so we put that possibility to bed. A massive cargo ship, one of 250-odd such mishaps, lay like a beached whale on the reef under the plane, rusted hollow and helpless, but as much a part of the reef now as the coral heads and fish that call it home. The waves closed out on the majority of the reef, but found form in deep passes. It was hard to tell what they were doing from the plane, but the potential was exciting.

## HIDDEN GEM

The island seemed dry at first, a bit like the islands east of Africa — Madagascar and Reunion and even a bit like Australia, but with the radical topography of Tahiti or Fiji. Despite being so close to Australia — 1400 kilometres — a dry brown landscape is where the similarities end.

'How can this place be so close to Australia and be so French?' Koby asked. I had done a little study on the flight on the way over and had learned that Captain Jimmy Cook discovered the island in 1774. He didn't do much with it, and in 1853 Napoleon III, looking for a strategic military base, moved in and the French have governed it since. In the same way as the English used Australia, the French sent their criminals there, who became known as 'Wretches in Paradise'. Now, the island's as French as frog's legs. Noumea, its capital, is like a ritzy beachside suburb in France, complete with nude sunbakers and Euro-style cafes. We spent three days on land and then boarded the boat with our three new friends, Yossi, Manu and Alexander. These three men, from different corners of the earth, summed up the place better than anyone.

'Yes, it is expensive,' said Manu in his apologetic English. 'But it is very beautiful.' Manu is a content local surfer, one of only fifty on the island. They generally only surf on weekends, taking their boats out to the break of choice for the day and leaving the line-up pretty empty for the majority of the week. 'We have three surfing clubs here, because we get three times the money from the government. Ha!' He has a laugh like a stretched rubber band that winds up and snaps out in one breath. Manu lives just outside Noumea and surfs the southern reefs on the western side of the island. 'Every reef pass has waves, but my favourite wave is Ouana.'

We went there the first afternoon of our boat trip. It's a left-hander that is offshore in the midday trades, and during that trip, our anchor touched the reef more than anywhere else on the whole trip. It's a long wrapping left-hander that we surfed from four to six feet, a cross between Reunion Island's St Leu and Desert Point in Indo. It wraps and builds for 200 metres as it heads into the pass and was one of the best waves I've ever surfed. And there was nobody there — there weren't even any sharks!

'This is bullshit!' barked Clint. 'Fuck!' The kid has so much energy and his rapid-fire and excitable mouth have earned him the nickname 'Tourette's'. The excited charger can't seem to get enough colour in his language without swearing uncontrollably. His surfing is just as energetic, but has been ironed out by the perfect points of the Gold Coast where he lives. He is a guy who goes hard in everything he does.

Our first surf got us thinking: why has nobody really come here before? How many waves are there? It was pumping. Basically, the island lifestyle has made the locals lazy, and as the weekend is their only surfing time, they have stuck to the waves they know. In the same way, Poto didn't surf Teahupoo until 1990. 'I had so many perfect waves out the front of my house,' he once told me. 'Why would I need to go looking?'

'There are also some reefs in the north that we haven't surfed yet,' said Manu, referring to the New Caledonian coast that slides northwest as if pointing to New Guinea. 'I have seen them when we go fishing, but have not surfed them yet.' It didn't seem to bother him, as hordes of other surfers haven't been forced to look further afield yet. Manu only had one rule, which he broke himself regularly: 'We have a circle and take it in turns for waves.'

I met two locals in the water one morning, one of whom was itching to find out if we liked the waves there. I told him we did, very much. They were very welcoming and the feeling in the water was great. I guess it always is when the waves are good. 'Yes I have been to the Gold Coast, to Kirra, and there are so many people,' the local said.

'That must frustrate you,' I commented as we sat out the back, in a circle, waiting for our own waves.

'No,' he replied. 'Because I know I'm coming back here.'

Joel was the standout that day, and after a couple of tips from Koby to get his bottom turns deeper, the kid went crazy. 'It's a bit scary surfing with guys at this level,' he told me. The former Aussie champ didn't realise he's at that level already and that he was just waiting for his confidence to catch up to his flowing ability.

Yossi, a surfer from Israel, has made Bondi his home — and New Caledonia his love. He was a hard worker. With his background of compulsory military service, he took much of the cooking and cleaning duties on himself while Manu kicked back with practised island ease. But it didn't cloud Yossi's appreciation of the place. 'I first came here four years ago,' he said. 'Just looking for some new spots. I knew there had to be waves here so I just flew here and looked through their yellow pages and started calling people, looking for surfers.' He found Manu, and they have been surfing buddies ever since. Since moving to Australia over five years ago, Yossi maintains a lifestyle that allows him to travel to New Caledonia at the drop of a hat for a new swell. He partners Manu in the surf charter business.

'There are so many good waves here and it's so close to Australia. It's amazing there are not more surfers.' Yossi is a smart man with a good business head. 'You just have to find something you love and try to make money out of it,' he told me. It sounded simple.

## THE CAPTAIN

Alexander was the captain of the boat *The Viking*, a fifteen-metre yacht that made him smile like a proud father. Though he changed them daily, he wore nothing but speedos the whole week. Every pair was blue, their fade proof of their age. Alexander was born in Austria and his strong body and accent soon earned him the nickname 'Arnie'. We had him recite 'I'll be back' all trip. Alexander lived in Australia for a couple of years in the late eighties before setting sail from Perth with the winds of fate and time on his side. New Caledonia was his retirement plan. The middle-aged bloke spoke four languages, but preferred to read English novels while we surfed.

'I like reading English. I think the language is better because it seems to only take one sentence to say what would take the German language about four sentences.' I asked why he had decided to live in New Caledonia and his answer was so simple it came without thinking.

'I lived one year in New Guinea, Fiji, Tahiti … but when I sailed to New Caledonia, it was like arriving in New York, but with the same beauty of any other Pacific island. You have everything you need here. If you want to buy a Ferrari, you can! If you want to buy any food, you can get it here! That's why it is the best island in the Pacific. It has everything.' He dropped his head back to his book. Alexander goes out every weekend with his French girlfriend when he's not steering a charter. He has a good life and the smile to prove it.

## THE WAVES

We surfed all day during a three-day swell that ranged from three to six feet before going flat. The surf was a mix of long rippable and barrelling lefts to short punchy rights, and it seemed as if we hadn't even touched upon the whole island. On the flat days we found adventure in spear fishing and snorkelling. The highlight was when Koby emerged from the water with a ten kilo lobster as long as himself. 'I was chasing this lobster down a rock shelf when the thing poked me in the eye. I shot the fucker right in the head.' It fed ten of us.

Koby takes pride in being the gnarliest guy in any line-up, or in any situation, whether it's floating over a dry reef, chasing sharks, or keeping the grommets in line. He is always the first or last to do something and it's in his nature to make an impact. He doesn't travel with soap or towels or wax, but brings cases of music and DVDs. He's more than willing to let you use, or even keep, anything of his — and he makes free use of your things in return.

'You've never met anyone like me,' he told Clint one day when he had pushed his cheeky antics just a little too far. 'I will tie you up and just watch you all day crying in the sun — just for fun!'

If you haven't seen Koby lately, it's because he's been growing muscles and tattoos, dating models and living in LA, breaking into Hollywood and teaching Paris Hilton how to surf. He's an unusual character, and leads an interesting life.

You get to know everyone pretty well on a boat trip. We got to know New Caledonia quite well too — but not well enough. Before leaving the boat, we checked the map for undiscovered passes, and plans were already in place for another trip.

As I flew west to my home on the biggest island in the world, all I could think about was the little island lost in the Pacific. How many more could there be, I wondered? It's a question every traveller faces at some stage. Do you finish exploring one place and really get to know it? Or do you keep looking for new places?

Captain Jimmy Cook may have left this place, but captain Alexander was staying put, and, after experiencing it myself, I kind of wanted to as well.

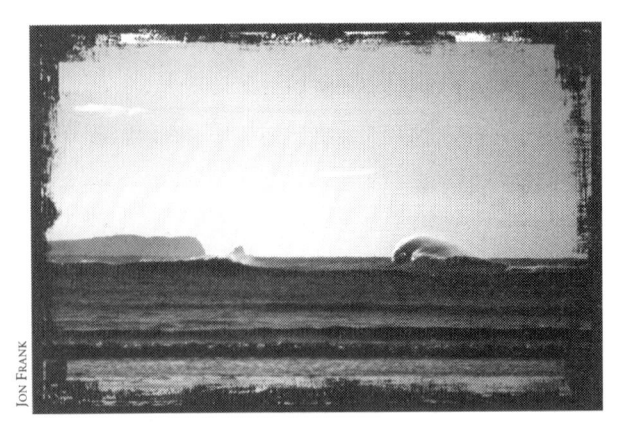

# NATIVE MYSTERIES
## NEW ZEALAND

'There are no native land mammals in New Zealand. None ….' Every now and then, there is a useless or interesting fact that momentarily consumes your interest. Since a wave hadn't come through for a few minutes, I was thinking about what my friend Fred had said in the line-up at Allen's Beach, deep in the South Island. My head ached from the several duck dives that had squashed ice cream between my ears; it was so cold I felt like icebergs were trying to move through my veins and my feet were struggling for feeling. Still my senses tingled from the view and I was warmed by the thoughts that surrounded me. I searched the big mountains for answers and they rose and fell into valleys and running rivers. It was a natural wonderland that made me feel as if I was surfing on the set of *The Lord of the Rings*. I was in a new place — and I was very interested.

Dunedin: May 2007. The sky was blue but the air was cold. It was almost winter and as the sun went down, the season became more obvious. First of all, some of the mountains were capped with snow which told me they were either very high, very cold, or both. There were no surfers around, except myself. Fred was watching from the beach, snow jacket on, walking her dog. The dog had a jacket on too. New Zealand has a very small population (4 million) — and out of that population, not many surf. Picture the geography and imagine the possibilities: 15,134 kilometres of coastline, open to every swell, protected from any wind.

If it's onshore on one side, it's not that far to drive to the other. And unless you're at the city beaches like Gisborne or Plymouth, or the perfect spots like Raglan, the only activity you'll find around you is cows and sheep munching on the vibrant green grass — and the farmers tending them.

Despite the fact that Dunedin is heavily populated and home to a youth culture with a growing sport and underground music scene, not many people surf there. I surfed by myself every day. The waves were really fun — beach break A-frames find shape up and down the whole beach. Since there were no surfers and every bank looked good, it was hard to know where to surf, so I moved around; this also helped fight off the cold. Cows and sheep watched me, the odd sea lion barked at me for invading his space and giant kelp clung to the nearby point, dancing with the tide.

The Maori named New Zealand Aotearoa, which means 'land of the long white cloud'. You don't have to hang out here long to realise why. Sometimes, the blanket of clouds seems as fixed as the landscape.

New Plymouth: April 2005. There was dew on the lush green grass, which sprawled into hills and down to the empty ocean. I was on a trip with Kieren Perrow and Matt Wilkinson, assessing the value of New Zealand as a potential Search WCT location. As we wandered down a hillside, Kieren called, 'Is the fence electric?' He was a little worried.

'Fuck, I don't know. Probably. Don't touch it!'

Off in the distance, strong lines were made crisp by the offshore breeze. A left peeled past the lonely point and, further out, a reef break barrelled left and right. There was no access to it. Between us and the beach, a distance of some 400 metres, was green pastureland; hills rolling down towards the shoreline, a few sheep and a bunch of cows.

'Are they bulls? Fuck!' Kieren might be from Byron Bay, but we don't know anywhere else in the world where the pastureland goes right to the shore like it does in New Zealand. We jumped the fence and ran to the surf, past the bulls that stamped their feet disapprovingly. Cows regarded us curiously and sheep fled as we made our way to the shore. We had to cross a river whose running water had smoothed the stones, but made them slippery for our cold feet. 'Ouch, that's freezing!' I said.

'Yeah, look where it's coming from,' said Kieren.

I looked behind me to where Mount Taranaki stood. It's a dormant stratovolcano, 2518 metres high — and it was so close that we could have walked there. Although it was not winter, snow was finding its way down half the symmetrical mountain, where it melted and entered the ocean. Judging by what my feet were telling me, the snow hadn't had time to warm in its journey down the mountain. It was incredibly cold, especially to my bare feet.

Mount Taranaki is a beautiful mountain. In fact, it is so symmetrical that film-makers exploited its similarities with Mount Fuji to create the movie *The Last Samurai*. Many rivers and creeks enter the ocean at its base, which creates the numerous reef breaks and beach banks. The whole coastline follows the symmetry of the mountain, making a semi-circled coastline, like a bay inverted.

As I've mentioned, if one side is onshore in New Zealand, you go to the other side. Depending on which side you are on, there are a series of left points or right points. The best of them is Stent Road. This is only accessible by car and therefore you'll find it hard to surf alone here. That's cool, though, because just looking up at Mount Taranaki leaves you feeling overwhelmed by nature. And if that's still not enough, all you have to do is run through a paddock to be alone — once you've got past the animals, that is. Just don't take a red board.

For some New Zealanders, getting to their local break is a little easier. For Daniel Kereopa, Raglan — the famous left-hand point — would have to be one of the best waves in the world. But for the 2007 National Champ and 2006 Aotearoa Maori champ, it's more than home. It's made him who he is and is part of what he is. His family owns most of the land around the point at Indicators, and because of this, and his surfing ability, he surfs the place with authority. Though most events and car parks are at Manu Bay, Indicators is where it starts. It's the best of the series of points that make up Raglan. On any given day you'll find Maui campervans parked on the point, waiting for it to clean up, or boards on the roof of cars in the nearby town of Hamilton. Raglan is the holy grail for surfers in New Zealand because of its Maori roots and its reputation. It is long and perfectly paced; after one glimpse you know that you've experienced something very special.

Sometimes, people from New Zealand do the haka. It's a tribal and cultural dance that is traditionally performed by Maoris before going into war and is meant to strike fear into their opponents. When I saw Maz Quinn do it for the first time, it was not very convincing. I mean no disrespect; Maz is just too shy. He keeps his explosive energy for surfing and displays his patriotism through a little green Kiwi necklace and a tattoo on his bicep.

'I lost my necklace once,' he said, showing me a small Kiwi on his arm. 'So I got a tattoo instead. I can't lose that.'

Maz's shyness on land is a contrast to his intensity when he is on a wave. The shy boy from Gisborne takes it to another level when he is in the water. It is obvious that he has learned how to dance with the ocean. Everyone who has seen Maz — and his explosive surfing — regards him as a true entertainer. No matter whether he is coming first or last, his surfing is big. It is no secret that he has underachieved, but everyone has different goals. 'At the end of the day, I just want to surf and for people to take notice,' he said. 'I don't want to be seen as a shit surfer. One of my main goals is to be known as a good surfer. If I can do that, I'll be happy.'

Right now, Maz is pretty happy. He's home — and what a place to break. The air here is fresh and the hills are a never-ending green, intersected by flowing rivers and creeks. It's almost like Australia — just condensed in colour and topography — and the inhabitants often argue that they fit more sports stars into their two small islands than Australia does on the biggest island continent on earth. New Zealanders definitely hold their own.

The beach at Maz's house is up there with the best. It is long and sandy, and riddled with deep channels and rip banks.

'I grew up here,' said Maz proudly. 'Right in front of Wainui Beach. It's like a little surf city. Everything here sort of revolves around the beaches. An hour or so either side is just endless reefs and points too, so you just need the right swell direction and there are perfect waves at our doorstep.'

This is not only Maz's favourite beach; he is also this beach's favourite surfer. He is a local hero. He even has a burger named after him in the main street — the 'Maz Burger'. Despite his love for his home beach, though, Maz loves nothing better than jumping in a car and travelling. It's one of the best things to do in New Zealand.

The landscape surprises you around every corner as the mountains are so big and green that you can't see very far ahead of you. There is one constant in the landscape — sheep. The fact that there are more sheep than humans in New Zealand reflects their small population, despite the fact that it is a cause of many Australian jokes. Nonetheless, sheep are everywhere. There are so many, in fact, that they have indented the steep hills with their foreign hooves as they climb higher for food.

'Dunedin is one of my favourite spots,' said Maz of the southernmost city in the southernmost island. 'They have the best waves. It's just really cold. I spend a lot of time down there in the summer. You can get away with a short arm steamer [full-length wetsuit] and there are so many crazy places if you know where to go.'

When Maz reached a certain age, he realised that the fresh solitude of New Zealand could only take him so far. To take his surfing to the next level, he had to move to Australia and subject himself to the best Aussie talent. Of course, he was the butt of the best Aussie jokes too. 'Yeah, I copped a bit. It's just the Aussie sense of humour though, so I didn't let it worry me.'

Despite being surrounded by talent in his hometown of Gisborne, with guys like Blair Stewart and Damon Guiness as his neighbours, Maz moved to Australia to contest the Australian junior series. This is without doubt the most competitive junior circuit in the world. Every winner of this junior series has gone on to rank among the top 20 in the world. And that was something Maz quietly had his eye on.

'I'd won a couple of Cadets and a few open titles, I think,' he said of his New Zealand career. The fact that Maz has a hazy memory of his early achievements shows that he has always aimed for excellence on a world scale.

'They've got a pretty good circuit there in New Zealand — eight or ten contests a year. The boardriders' scene in Gisborne is active as well, which helped a lot. But I knew that if I wanted to get anywhere, I had to come to Australia and do well on the junior series. So I lived in Sydney for eight months and did the junior series full on for about three years.'

Maz developed very close friendships with a lot of the Australians, who played on his shy character and fed off his explosive talent. Jake Patterson, Ozzie Wright and Sam Carrier all spent a lot of time with him. Maz also came to Australia at a time when the junior series was incredibly competitive, with surfers such as Danny Wills, Will Lewis, Jay Phillips, Chris Davidson and Luke Hitchings. Maz worked hard to beat these guys and eventually, in his last year, all his hard work paid off. He won. 'It was my last year so I was pretty stoked,' he said.

At that stage, Maz was spending a lot of his time in Oz competing. But once he started on WQS he began going home again. The fresh air, surrounding mountains and endless rip banks called for him. So did the taste of the 'Maz Burger'.

'Just being in Australia was so good, because you can go to any beach and there will be at least ten stand outs, where at home there is only one or two. So the standard was definitely higher and it improved my surfing a lot.'

Of course, qualifying for the 2001 WCT made Maz a national hero. All of a sudden, the shy boy had to talk. He's getting better at it, but I'd imagine it's improved about as much as his Haka.

Hawaii

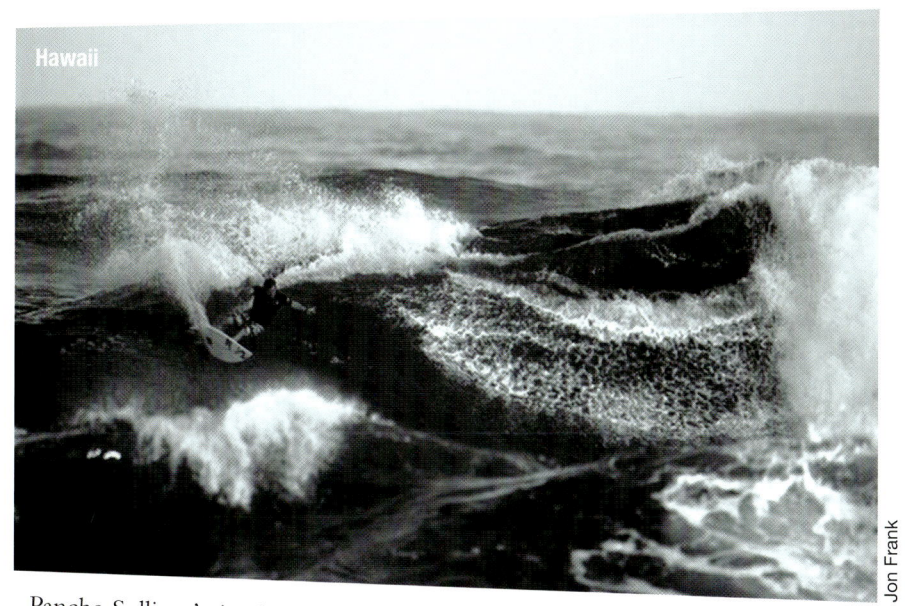

Jon Frank

Pancho Sullivan's timeless manhandling of the Hawaiian power. Here, he makes his way through the Haleiwa bowl.

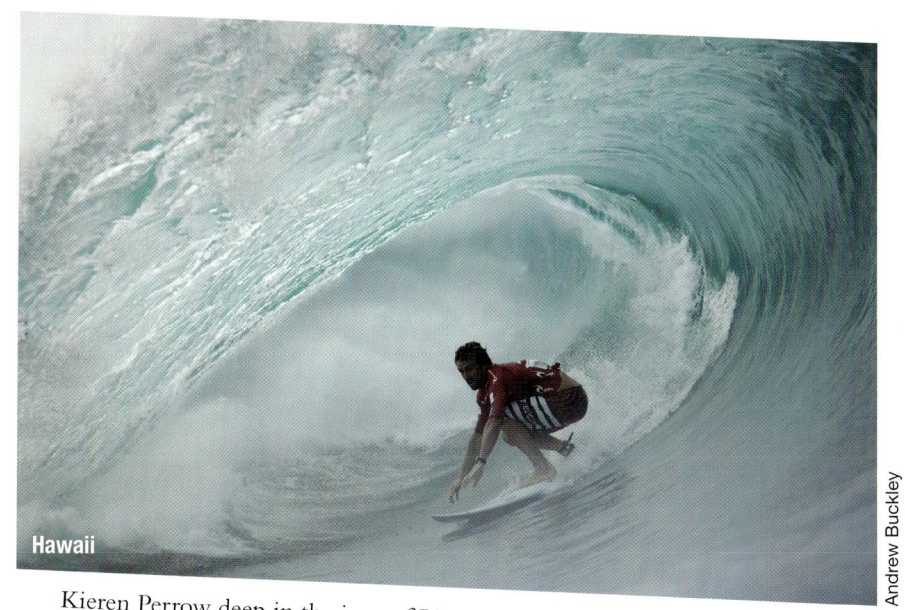

Hawaii

Andrew Buckley

Kieren Perrow deep in the jaws of Pipeline.

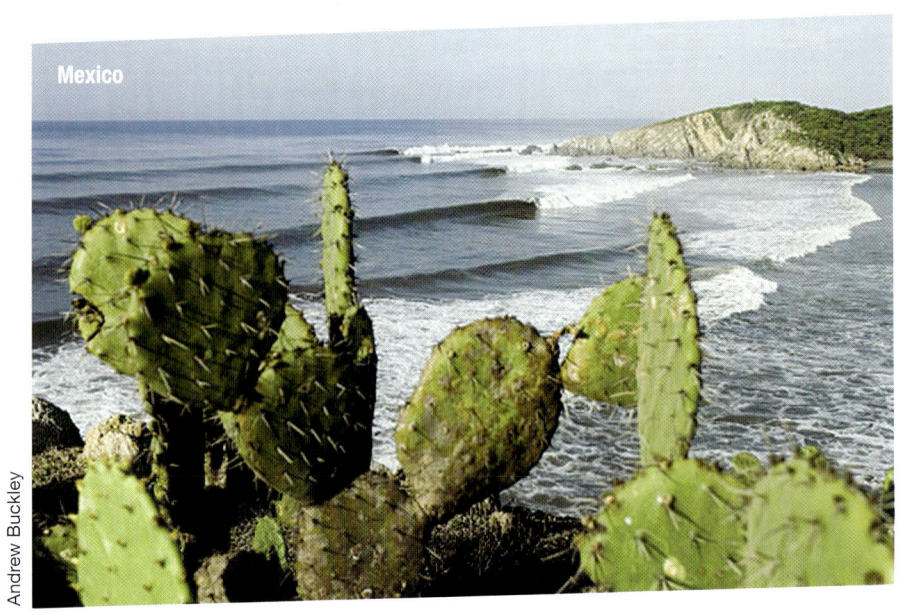

Mexico can look like this around every corner.

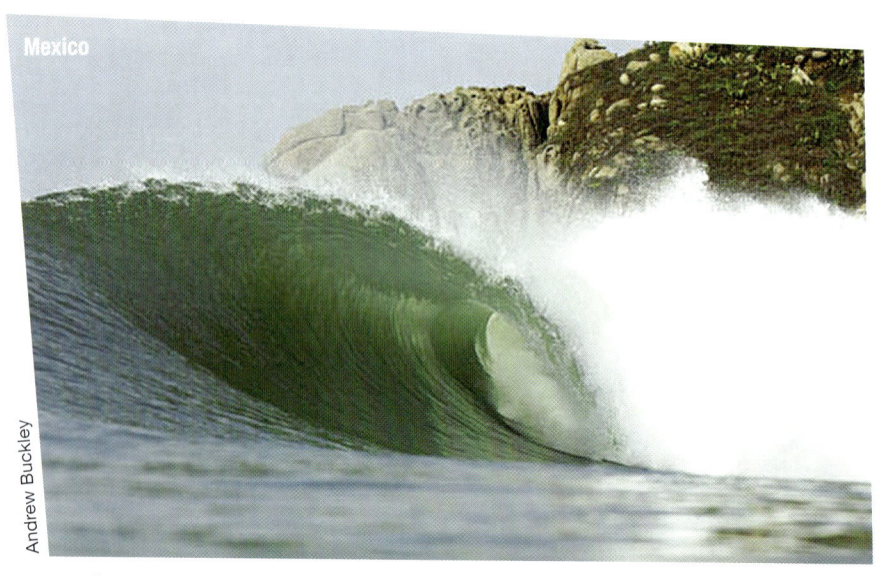

The site for the Rip Curl Search WCT produced perhaps the best waves ever witnessed in competition. This shot must have been taken in a heat, as there were no waves going unridden in free surfing sessions.

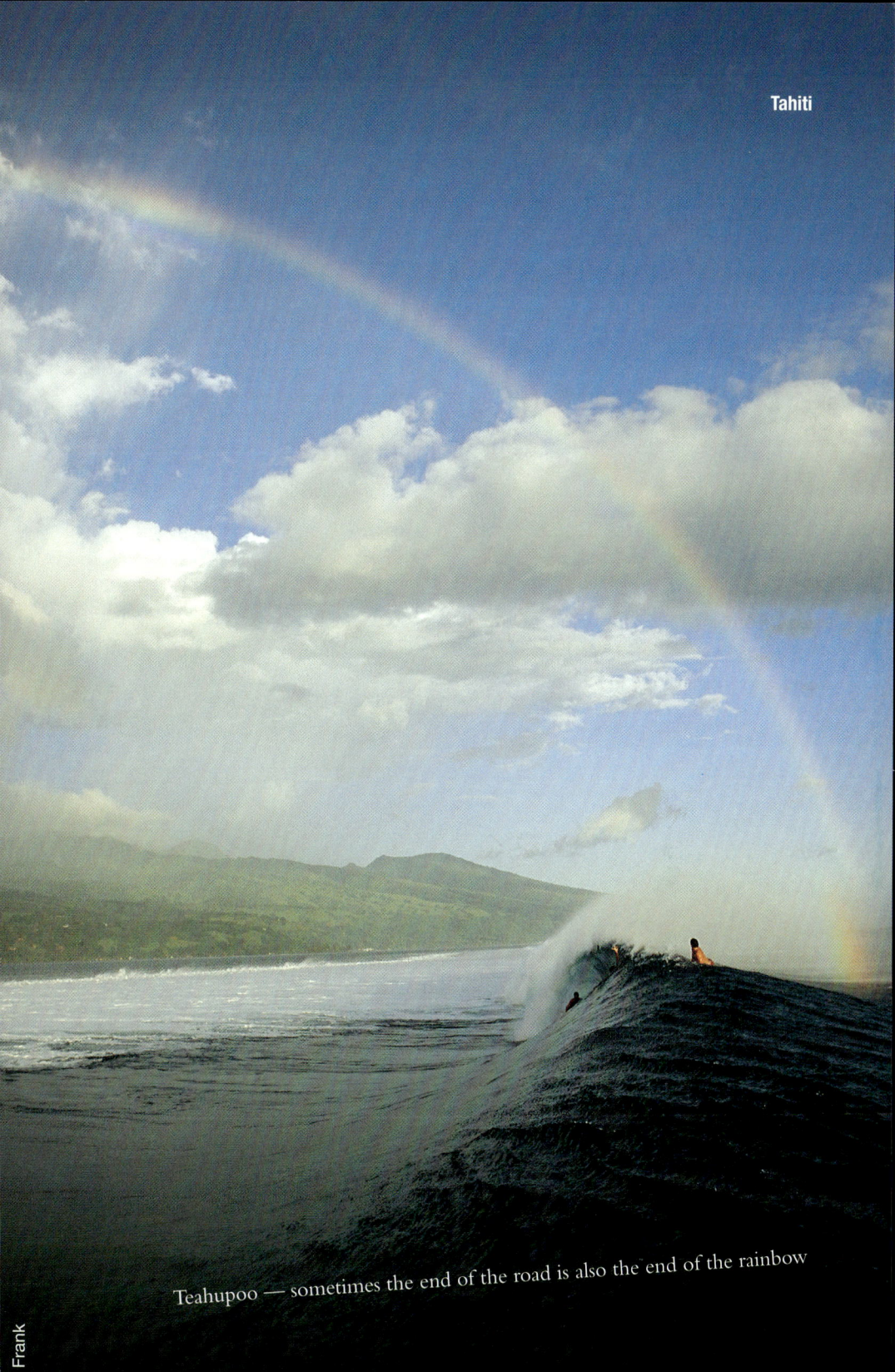

**Tahiti**

Teahupoo — sometimes the end of the road is also the end of the rainbow

Frank

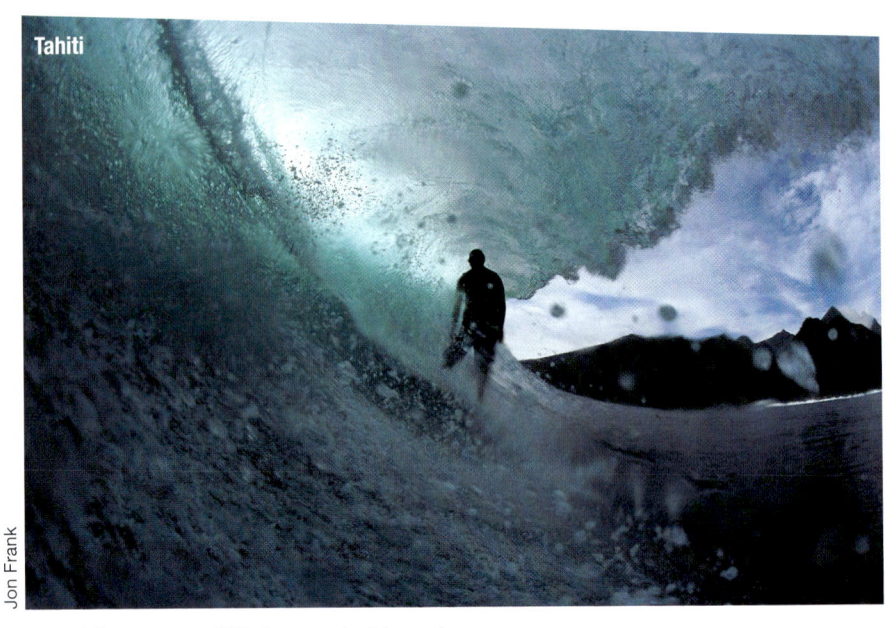

The power of Teahupoo, inside and out.

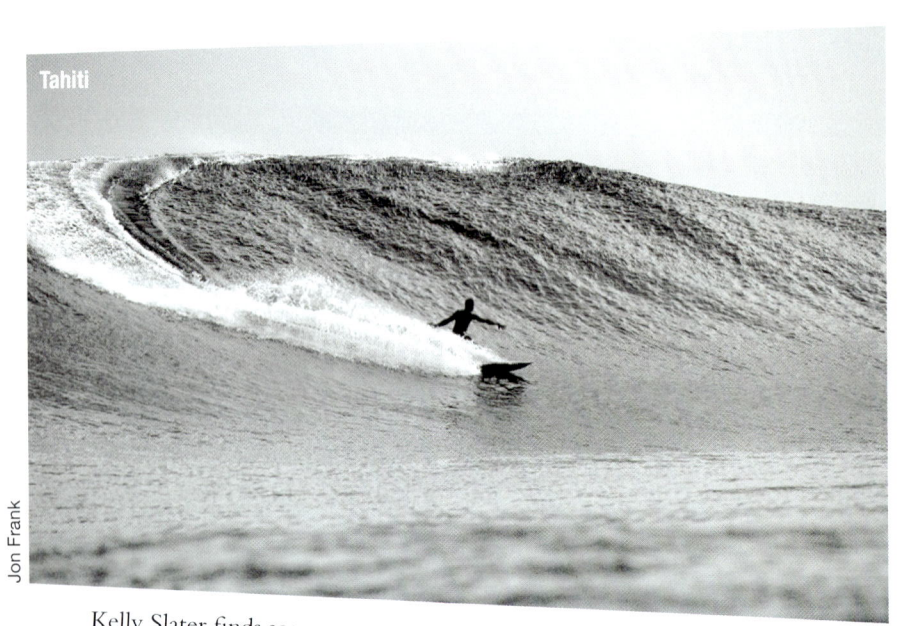

Kelly Slater finds some room to move, towing in to an outer Pacific bommie.

An aerial view of 'The Superbank', from Snapper to Kirra. Since the inception of the sand-dredging project, some Gold Coast surfers have covered this distance in one wave.

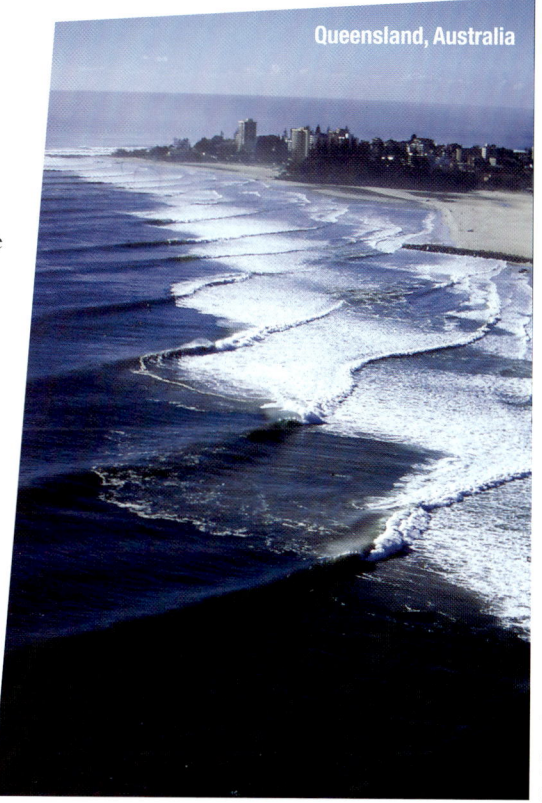

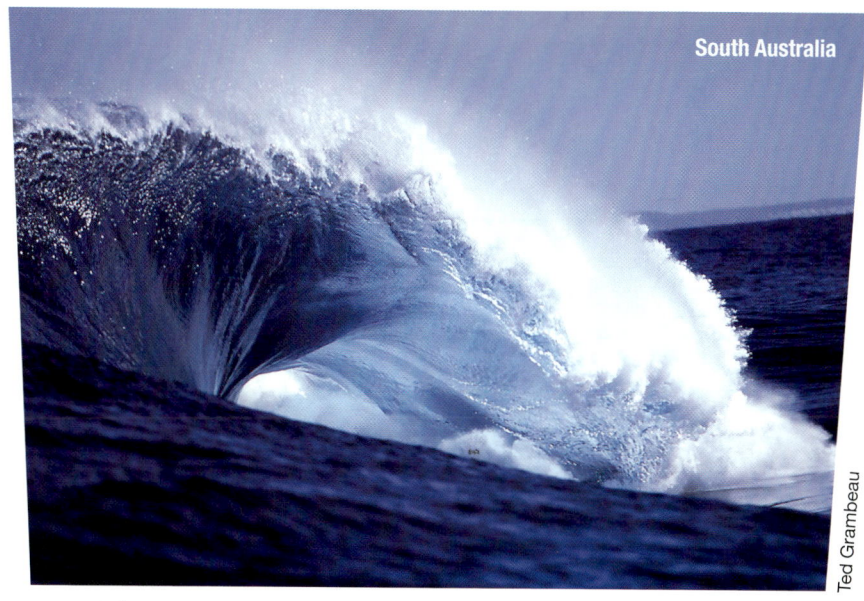

The raw ocean power of Cyclops, South Australia.

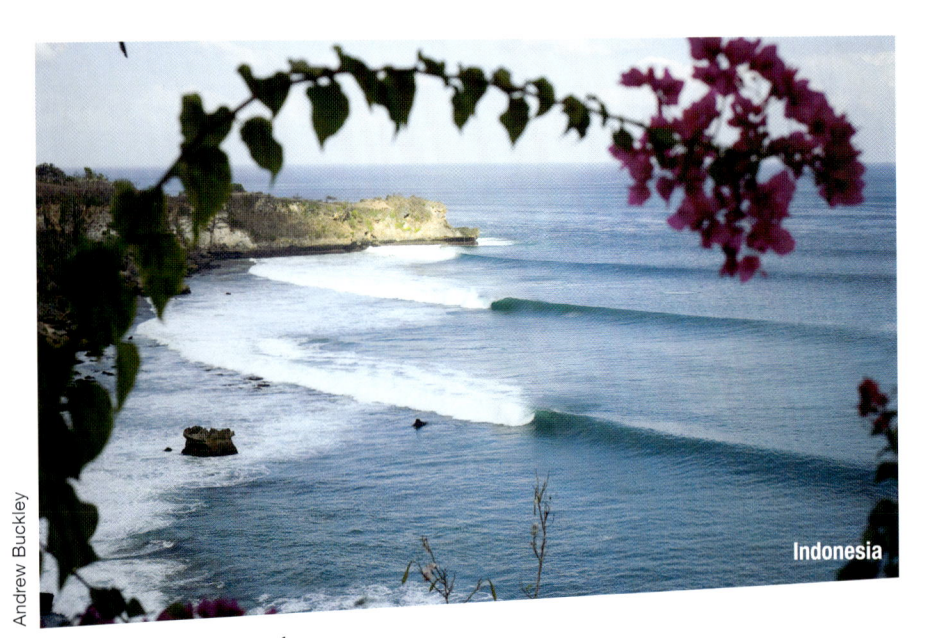

Occy's Left in Sumba.

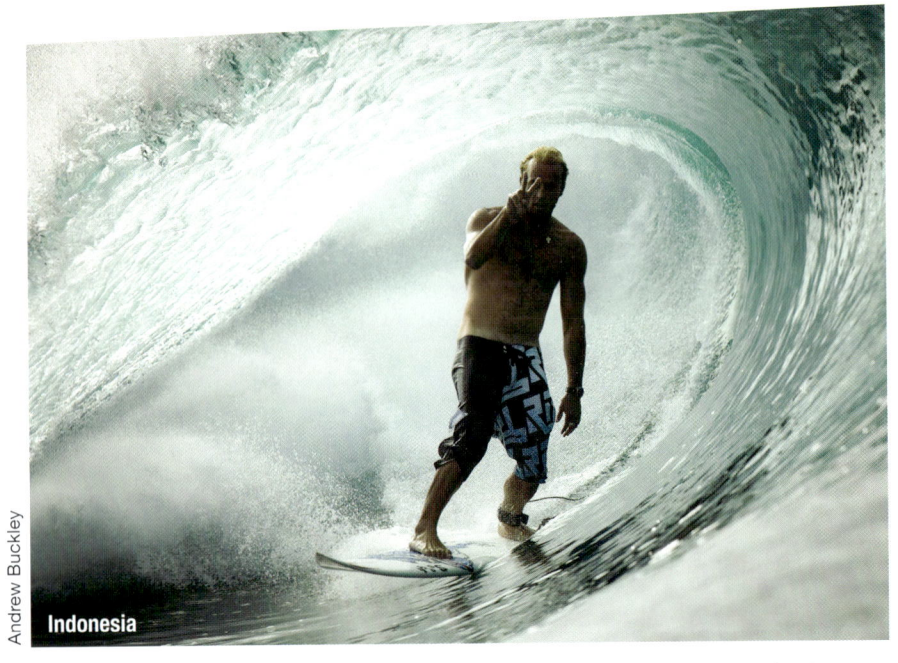

Nathan Hedge, locking in to a new discovery in the Mentawai Islands.

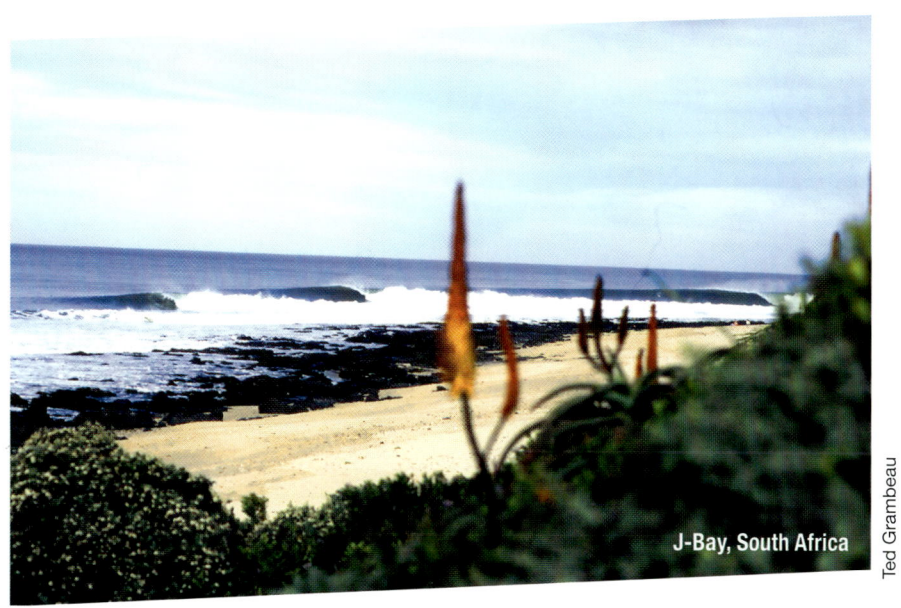

The lines at Jeffreys Bay are enough to hypnotise anyone.

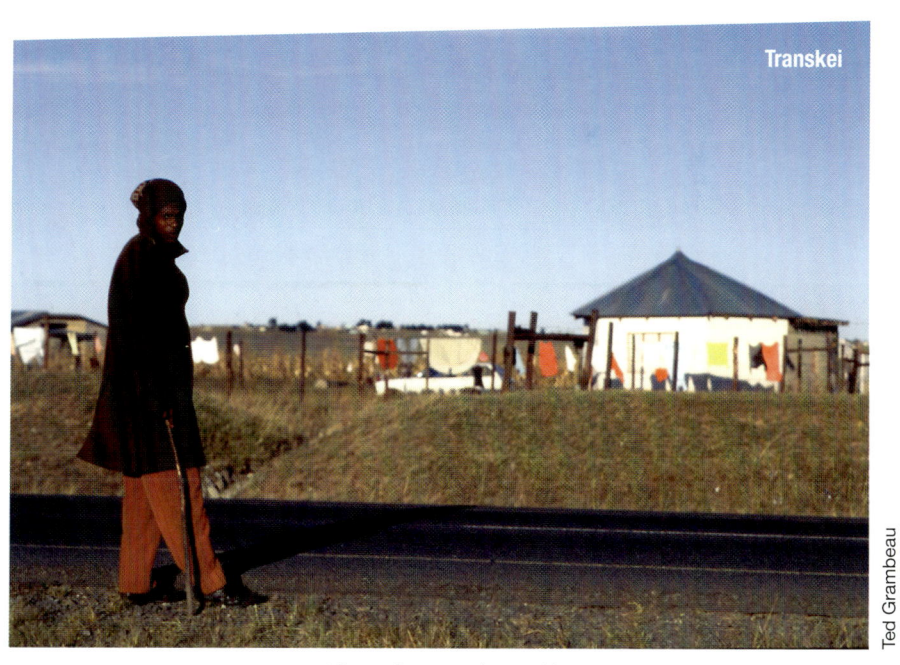

Life in the Transkei is like no other in Africa.

**Reunion Island**

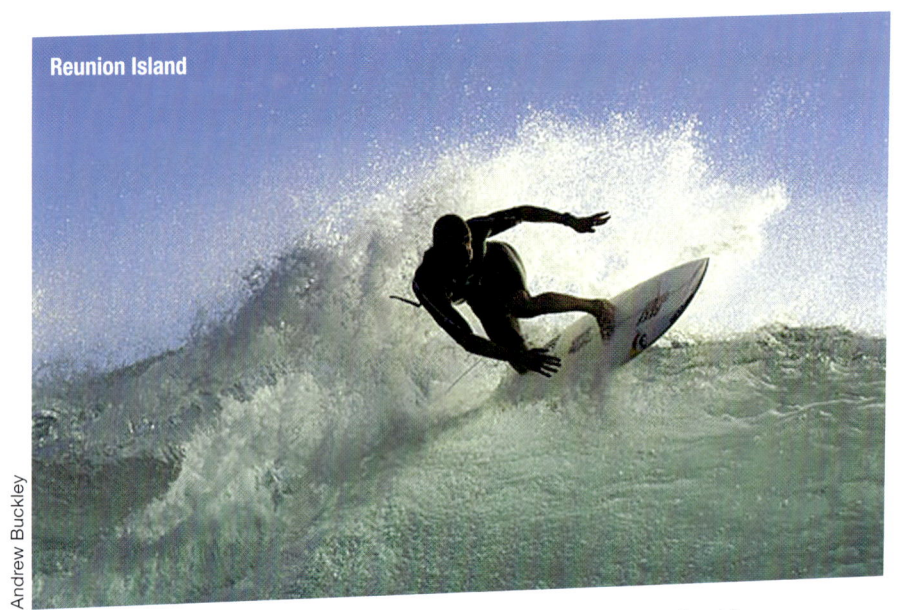

Mick Fanning glides above the lipline at St Leu. Reunion Island has an amazing marriage of French and African cultures ... and one of the most high-performance waves in the world.

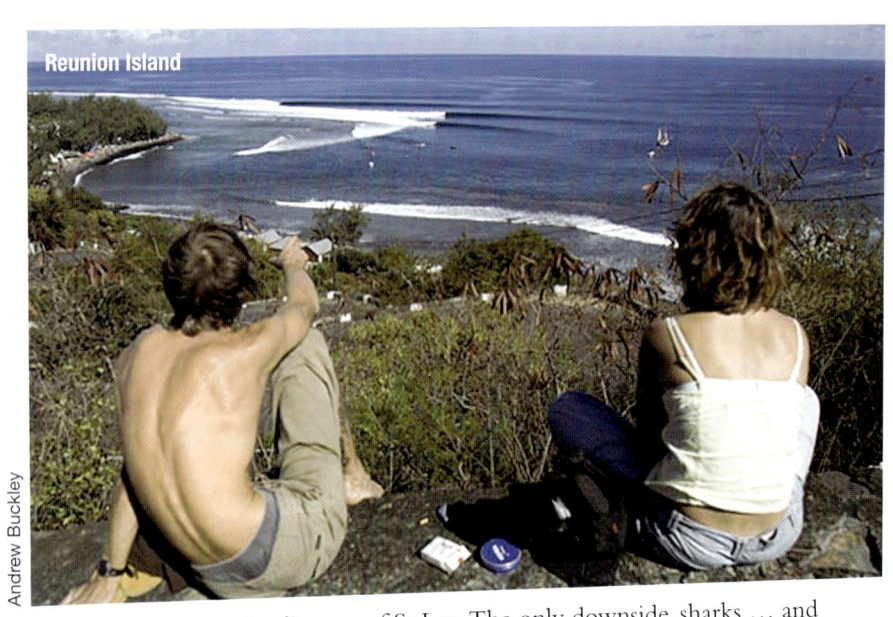

**Reunion Island**

The perfect wrapping line-up of St Leu. The only downside, sharks ... and lots of them.

'Yeah, they were sort of picking up on it [the fact that Maz was going to qualify] after each result I got. I was getting emails and phone calls from everyone at home, especially the media. Then when I made it, it was crazy. Every TV show, radio station — they all picked up on it. It was good. I've sort of learned how to deal with it. It can only boost your career so …'

More than anything, though, his win was a boost for New Zealand surfing. The small country in the south Pacific had another export, another attraction apart from the landscape. It had another sporting hero.

'Hopefully my winning can show any New Zealand grommy that they can make it. I hope that my making it pushes the other guys. I'm sure I won't be the last New Zealander to qualify. I'm sure Bobby Hansen and my brother will qualify and do it for New Zealand as well.' I'm sure his younger brother will too.

His name is Jay. And with a world junior title already under his belt, a residential stint in Australia and a certain inconsistency, it looks as if he is well on the way to following in Maz's footsteps. His time will come. We all know that.

'Yeah, he sort of is like me,' said Maz. 'As soon as he switches his free surfing to contest surfing he'll take off.'

They are both winning New Zealand events, but still underachieving on a world scale. In any case, Maz and his brother have added two more sports heroes to the Kiwis' proud heritage, just as Daniel has gained fame for the indigenous Maoris. Maybe they will inspire a whole new generation of Kiwi surfers. Maybe the long, cold beach breaks and points of New Zealand will one day be crowded with more than just sheep, cattle, running rivers and a ruggedly beautiful topography.

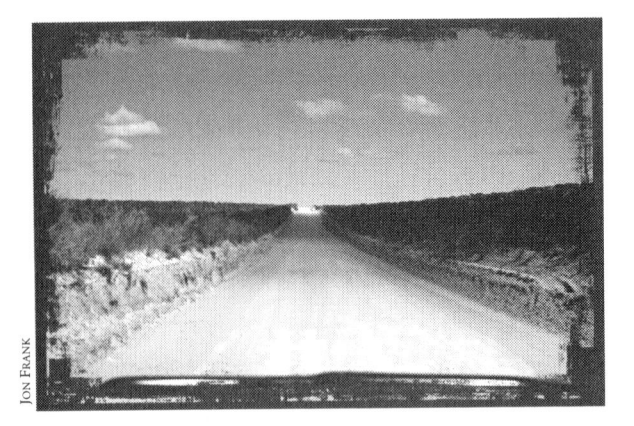

# THE SOUTHERN CROSS OVER
## AUSTRALIA

Bondi Beach, 2.30 pm, 5 January 2008. The sky was blue, but it felt and burnt red. It was crowded, with not too much spare sand to lay your towel, let alone place your surfboard. The lifeguard patrol led the beach like moving statues in an outdoor museum. They were putting on a show for their new reality TV show. The reality is: people burn, drown, get stung, eaten and robbed (mostly by seagulls) here — all worthy TV subjects — and the lifeguards stood in front of the waves that had travelled as far as the tourists. The difference is, the waves have been coming here a lot longer. It was this minority of foreigners, who had simply borrowed the beach and the culture for the day, that the lifeguards were watching. Soon, someone would be stuck in a rip, or have a bluebottle wrapped around his or her arm, or swear they'd seen a shark. The surfers out the back were used to this and were more than likely better ocean-goers than the lifeguards. They surfed in and out of the flags ... wherever the wave took them.

In the line-up, a grommet kicked out in the shore break and the wave rolled in to shore. There, it splashed the feet of a one-year-old baby. The baby already knew how to float safely and swim back to his mother. The waves made him giggle. In Australia, you learn to swim before you learn to walk. On the sandy beach behind me, the first layer of beachgoers began yet another day of bronzing under a sun that statistically delivers more skin cancer than anywhere in the world. (If you ever want to pick out an Australian, just look for freckles and sun-damaged skin.) The smell of sunscreen and the sound of seagulls floated in the salt air of the freshening northeast sea breeze. Behind the beach, the new Australians, mainly ethnic communities, contradicted the Australian culture and picnicked on the grass (for some reason, the majority don't like sand), while across the road the traffic of humans crossed the road back to the beach with melting ice creams, umbrellas and surf craft of every variety. It was just another day at Bondi Beach, but for the core surfing community of Australia, there were 7097 other beaches where they'd rather be.

## SURFERS PARADISE

Perfectly groomed point breaks, warm, crystal-clear water, the solitude of the sub-tropical hinterland ... It's a place where government officials and businessmen sit on a board — both at work and at play — and where a council played God and pumped sand to Snapper Rocks, creating a wave that actually displaced another man-made phenomenon — Kirra — as the world's best point. However, in doing so, it joined the dots of all the points into a Super Bank. Wet and Wild, Planet Hollywood, Movie World, Hard Rock Cafe ... what do you want to do? A $500 piece of sushi or a meat pie for $2? What do you feel like? A beer on Cavil

Avenue, a look at the strippers, a tequila — let's go mad! Where shall we stay? On a man-made island, in the tallest building in the southern hemisphere, or in a house on the beach? The wind is southerly — where shall we surf? Shall we go to Kirra, Snapper, Burleigh …? Or get away from the crowds and surf down the coast or at Palmy Beach or Mermaid? Make a decision, or don't — it doesn't matter. It will all be there again tomorrow at Surfers Paradise.

It was a hot day, like most. The UV rays burnt my skin as though there was a magnifying glass somewhere between the sun and Snapper Rocks, and my eyes had to squint for refuge. Funny thing was, it was 4.30 am! The sun had just popped over a pink horizon, and lit a line-up of perfectly groomed waves writing poetry upon water so clear that you could see the sand waving in formation all the way down to Kirra for another day's work. A crowd not unlike that at a huge sporting event jockeyed for position, thousands panning and sifting through the sand for their own piece of the Gold Coast.

Mmmm, where to paddle out from? The good thing about Snapper is, if you have never surfed here before, there will be about a thousand people paddling out before you. So you can always follow. But the ironic thing here is, the majority are actually kooks. So you may see some funny stuff — rock jumps, back wash demolitions and indecision — before someone like Mick Fanning or Joel Parkinson will come and show you how it's really done. But they do it so fast, you'd better pay attention, because you won't keep up. It's the same in the line-up. If you can't keep up, you'll be left behind, dropped in on, snickered at and glanced at with a look that says; 'If you are just getting in the way, you shouldn't be out here!' But everyone wants a crack at the Super Bank — and even the locals understand that.

I've seen people laugh, I've seen people cry. I've seen someone come in with three broken fins on a brand new board before they even caught a wave. I've seen surfers change from total disillusionment to pure elation after catching the best barrel of their life and getting their own piece of Surfers Paradise. I've seen kooks who can barely hold a line going across the wave and getting barrelled for a few seconds. People from up and down the Australian coast who come here for their annual holidays, talk stories over a beer in the surf club, while replays of the day's surfing run on the plasma screen in all corners of the room and surfing brand ads invade your attention. If you have come for surfing, you will find a place that has swallowed itself entirely. But if you want to escape — and you will — it's all there for you.

'You have to get away,' said Wayne 'Rabbit' Bartholomew (Bugs), a former world champion who has caught more waves on the Gold Coast than anyone. 'It's all so consuming down there at Cooly. I just love going back to my little shack in the hinterland.' Bugs, like most locals, balances the rush with a bit of solitude only fifteen minutes' drive away.

'I could never live amongst it either,' said Mick Fanning, who is a few hills back in geography and solitude. 'It's too hectic.'

You find most of its residents share the same view. It's a great place to go, but a great place to leave. And there is no better place with which to contrast the madness of the Gold Coast than the serenity of its hinterland.

Thousands of years ago, Mount Warning, the core of a huge and ancient volcano, spat a boiling load of rock all over the Gold Coast. You can see the lava rocks lining the points of Burleigh especially. Mount Warning is the first point of land to see sunlight on the east coast of Australia and the first place people go for a taste of nature. On the drive inland, you start to breathe a slightly more chilled air within fifteen minutes, as the caldera (bigger than the Gold Coast itself) fills with rich soil and ancient trees from the Jurassic era. Rivers run down its valleys where Aborigines once flourished around the high-energy mountain. In the local language it is called Wollumbin, which translates as 'cloudcatcher'. And there are plenty of stories of walkers, keen to see a sunrise, leaving in the early hours of the morning to march the two to three hours north (straight up) to get the first glimpse of the sun, only to be disappointed. Because even on clear days, the cloudcatcher lives up to its name.

In a country where people are used to driving for a few hours just to check the surf, the Gold Coast is one of the few places that contains everything in such a small area. One minute you are driving down from Mount Warning, watching cows in green pastureland; the next, you're amongst a boiling pot of surf culture on a beach so hot that even walking on it can sometimes give you third-degree burns on your feet.

Snapper Rocks can be quite a zoo — and as such it inspires a certain animalistic behaviour in its patrons. This is what the Snapper Rocks species looks like, from head to toe. He has blond hair, bleached by endless days in the sun and dried by hours in the wind and salt. The skin is freckled, probably peeling and wrinkling from an environment that is more or less an aging chamber. By the time he is thirty, he looks forty, but by the time he's forty, he looks sixty. Before he has left school, he has already had two sunspots burnt off his lip, and a suspicious mole taken from his freckled and marked back. His shoulders are broad, his arms gorilla-like, his lower back sore. It only takes a couple of years of paddling these points against a sweep which can be like paddling up Niagara Falls to acquire an upper topography built for speed and paddling endurance.

He has a tattoo: the Southern Cross, or some pattern of a rebellious nature. The boardies are long and beneath them are balls rashed from running back around the points, or maybe a suspect sexual encounter. He rides a Darren Handley or a Jason Stevenson surfboard. And by night, the girls ride him. He wagged many days of school to surf and probably left early. If he isn't a professional surfer, he has a job that is surf-friendly. Maybe he works in a bar, a hotel (the hospitality industry is huge) or does some kind of shiftwork (usually at Cooly airport) to accommodate his thirst for surfing all day every day. He lives fast, surfs fast and talks slow: 'Waves are pretty good today, eh! Whadda ya reckon … and that.'

But here, although their wave count and presence in the line-up wouldn't suggest it, the locals are the minority. Japanese escape their own social pressures of working eight days a week in Tokyo by coming to the Gold Coast, bleaching their hair blond and swearing occasionally. Brazilians have come in with the new tide on student visas, in large numbers and always in groups. They fit in with the Australian lifestyle as it is not unlike their own beach lifestyle back in Brazil. But it generally takes them a while to chill their passionate decibels and learn that all but the locals take turns. Their girls have sprinkled the sand in a beautiful display of womanhood that makes every run-around just a little bit slower and more interesting — it all adds to the full-on nature of the Goldy. This is a place where surfing never sleeps; where, during the night, sand is pumped to groom her banks for the next day's work while people party in preparation. And all the time new planeloads come in, adding to and subtracting from the spectacle that is the full-on surf town called Surfers Paradise.

## SURFING NATION

Snapper Rocks is where it all goes down. The sun comes over the horizon and provides a peek at what is now referred to, thanks to a sand-dredging project, as 'The Super Bank'. It is barely light and there are already fifty guys out, fifty guys waxing their boards, fifty guys on their way — and fifty more hitting the snooze button on their alarms. The sun is bright, the water is turquoise, the sand is gold, and in the background the high-rises of Surfers Paradise show the coast's true angle. People are moving — and it's all towards the surf.

While an astounding 11 per cent of the Australian population surf (according to Sweeney Sports Report 2002/2003), it seems that around 98 per cent of the population of the Gold Coast do. By 4.30 am, the sun has been up for twenty minutes and there are at least 150 people battling for the long waves that barrel, spit and reform all the way down to Kirra, at least two kilometres away.

Amongst them are former world champ Mark Occhilupo, Luke Egan, Joel Parkinson, Mick Fanning, Josh Kerr and Dean Morrison. If they were surfing anywhere else in the world, they would stand out like dog's balls. But in Australia, they are simply five more rippers in the water. In Australia, nobody gets treated like royalty. To get a wave out here, you have to be at this level, otherwise you'll only catch scraps. Hierarchy is decided by skill, not size. And, like the beaches, it is enforced and protected.

If you were raised on the Gold Coast as a surfer, you were raised to compete. Whether you want to or not, it's the only way you'll get waves. It's places like Snapper that inspire surfers and set the performance benchmark for new generations. These places are the reason the Gold Coast is leading the charge. Of Australia's seven world champions, three are from the Gold Coast — and, with Mick and Joel at the helm, there will be more.

'Joel and Dean are the whole reason behind my success,' said current world champion, Mick Fanning. 'Growing up, they were always better than me — and I wanted so badly to beat them, or be as good as them. If it wasn't for them, I wouldn't be where I am today.'

Along the rest of Australia's 25,760 kilometres of coastline lie more reasons for success. Like Australian swimmers, surfers win because Australia has the luxury of good facilities. Add to that a culture that prides itself in — and pours money into — its sporting stars, and they are riding a tidal wave of opportunity. All you have to do is not fall off. And if you do, somebody else won't, which is the essence of the real driving force behind Australia's competitiveness. That's one side of surfing in Australia — competition, performance, perfect waves, crowds. But it's not the only side.

## WILD WEST

There's an eerie feeling here. The land is untouched, except perhaps by ghosts. Three hundred and seventy-eight years ago two white men were cast ashore here after months of mutiny, murder and betrayal aboard a Dutch ship on its way to the Indies, present day Indonesia. What became of them, only the Aborigines know. I'd been warned about the ghost coast before I came, but as I sat on top of the red bluff, overlooking the Batavia Coast in Western Australia where their ship had run aground in 1629, I could hear the ghosts creeping between the wind roaring under the waves. I was sixty metres above sea level and miles from civilisation, looking out over an ocean and desert that's been neglected by all, even history.

Below me, a rare perfect left found form in an otherwise inhospitable coastline. It exploded onto the jagged reef and wrapped around the feet of the bluff, finishing where most water does — in the desert. The ancient shells and sandy beach of a protected bay became the mysterious border where the desert met the sea, of where life met death. Nathan Hedge was fishing off the cliff below me. I watched him wrestle a fish to shore, only to have it eaten by sharks. Out to sea, countless whales looked like a floating archipelago, breaching and bumping up in the crystal clear water. The ocean was alive.

But behind me, life stopped and the desert began, flat and endless. It was like looking into space on a clear night. Besides the occasional kangaroo or emu, the only life came from stubborn little bush shrubs, made evil by the action of the wind and the absence of shade. I had a 360-degree view, with nothing between the horizon and me. Just space, dead and flat. From my elevated position on the cliff I could see for the first time in my life the curve of the earth as it stretched away into a sphere. Out here, even the earth seems small. A bird flew below me, past the skeletal remains of an emu, and over the fossils of hundreds of shells, talismans of the last ice age, or perhaps the one before that. I was looking at a coast ignored by sailors. Dirk Hartog discovered the west coast of Australia in 1616 (162 years before James Cook) and thought it too inhospitable to land. It is a place with more shipwrecks than landings, a place where only the most hardened of surfers and fishermen venture. A place where women turn into men — such is the masculinity of the place — and even the flowers are wild. A place where, if you run out of petrol, you can die. And if you're there long enough, you'll surely go crazy. I watched the wave roll into shore and like everything else here, die in the Australian desert, empty and forgotten, except by surfers.

Hartog was the first to come to the desert. He was on his way to the Indies and landed near Shark Bay. He looked around a bit, and, finding nothing of interest, nailed a pewter dish to a tree to record his visit and left. He never came back. But George Simpson did. I met George in the car park of a local fishing spot; he is a 50 year old with muscles and a jawline as square and hard as the desert horizon. He first came in 1976. 'That wasn't here, though; that was down the coast a bit. A mate of mine was working on one of those stations when he found this wave.' His mate had discovered a perfect left and the next year he brought a surfboard. But according to George, it was a baptism of fire. 'He was surfing it by himself for a while, but with all the feeding frenzies going on around him, he freaked out!' That's when he called George, a surfer/fisherman from Yallingup who has lived his life by and around the sea.

'He wanted a surfing buddy, but it was hard to surf back then,' said George, 'because we were on single fins and these big fat boards. We just couldn't keep up with the wave.'

George, a competitive surfer at the time, had found an awesome watering hole in the desert. He didn't even realise there were more perfect oases in the area, places that would later ensure that this area was featured in special events and surfing movies. George has seen it all and, since that first year, has been camping out here every year.

Waves come from chaos: winds, storms, thunder and lightning. By the time they reach the desert, they are clean and free. Surfers come here for the same reason: to get away from the chaos of their lives and become simple again. Sam Hansen's been coming here for over a decade. 'I love it here,' he admitted. 'It's so alive; big fish, big waves, big whales. It's got the best of the ocean in every way.' The ability to catch fish goes a long way up here, especially as fresh fruit and vegetables rot within a few days, leaving you with just canned goods — unless you want to drive two hours to the corner store. 'I used to come up here for a few months at a time, but I've got the family now, so it's a bit harder to stay that long.'

The Hansens weren't the only family there. Small kids were everywhere, getting dirty in the cleanest possible way. The camp holds around forty to fifty people: some fishermen, some surfers, a few families, and the occasional old couple on their way around Australia in a campervan. You get to know everyone quite quickly and nobody stays too long. The desert is swift at killing things, or at least driving you crazy.

Day after day I watched a small peewee bird fly into its own reflection on the camp station's 4WD. I'm not sure whether it thought it was another bird, whether it was fascinated by its own reflection, or whether it had just gone crazy. It summed up the place pretty well.

There are no mirrors here; beards start growing and dirt congregates. You start to wonder, and question. Before you know it, you look in the rear-view mirror to put on some sunscreen and you can't recognise the face staring back at you. There is nothing to do here but surf. And if there is no surf, there is nothing to do but go crazy. The people who have come here the most often seem to have it down, growing raw and wild, like the surrounding landscape. To sit out in the line-up and watch someone paddle out wearing only a big beard and an old pair of stubbies and charge into a twelve foot set is not uncommon. You see it every day. Maybe the full moon keeps the fish away, or maybe that's when the sharks come out, or the craziness. I'm not sure, but there are some fishermen around here who charge harder than I've seen. Then, they'll disappear with the swell.

'It's considered one of the best fisheries in the world,' said George. He owns a few trawling boats and talks of times when his entire family have been stuck on a bit of reef with nobody within 2000 kilometres. Of taking Simon Anderson surfing here when he was seventeen. Of swimming through croc-infested rivers and chasing barramundi in the Kimberley. 'Mate, I remember one time being up there — you're fishing in these rivers where crocs and sharks are hanging out. This one time I was teasing a croc with this barra I had caught. We were fishing in a ten-foot tinny. All of sudden, this thing [a shark] about twenty feet long jumped out of the air, with half its body landing in the tinny. It froze for a second, off balance, and then slipped back in with the fish.'

This is a guy who sees sharks every day, while we watch the big tuna they're chasing diving out of the water, wondering what's happening. He even told us about the box jellyfish that stung him when he was bringing up the nets of his trawler. 'They fucking hurt, mate. But you get used to them. They don't kill you — that's a myth — but they'd probably kill a baby.'

'How big was the shark?' I asked about his earlier experience.

'I don't know — bigger than me.'

'Mate.' Hog jumped into the air. 'If Georgey boy says it's that big …' He made a circle with his arms. This time, his hands didn't meet, making a shark the size of his Landcruiser. We all agreed it was around six metres.

The desert is dead and lifeless; it's so thirsty it even drinks your piss. But the ocean is alive with possibilities. 'Put it this way,' George said.

'The first time I came to Gnarloo, it was three foot and high tide. I didn't surf it again for three years. What a mistake that was! I've seen thousands of kilometres of coastline here of line-ups that look exactly like that, but it's never been on a good day. When it's eight foot, high tide and offshore, I'm here. So who knows what's happening everywhere else?'

We split one day to find some waves, spending hours, then days, in our rented Landcruiser. I'd developed an interest in 4WDs of late and according to the local population, they are the only vehicles that don't fall apart.

The coast looked the same forever — and most of the reef is relentless, with rare opportunities for waves to break perfectly. In fact, the waves were as jagged and straight as the reef they closed out on. We were starting to sound like Dirk Hartog. After hours of searching and driving through a terrain yet to have a road, we found it. A right-hander too! The look on Kieren's face summed it up. It was dangerous, but perfect. A small opening in a small reef on a straight coastline. We spent two days and three nights camped on top of a hill in the middle of nowhere, surfing the wave of our dreams.

Back at camp a few days later, George had us around for a barbecue. We told stories about the desert, about the whales, about the bird flying into the mirror, about the two men who had murdered almost their entire ship in 1629, and we ate fresh fish. 'It's got that eerie feeling here, hasn't it,' confirmed George. Someone had done a shop run and brought back a paper and some news. 'A bomb went off in Jakarta today! Did you hear about it?'

George thought about the question and then looked at the questioner, then at the desert. In a place as far away from civilisation as you can get, even further away from its murderous history, you couldn't feel safer. 'Good to be up here, isn't it?' said George, as he walked back towards the fire.

## THE ANIMAL

The Australian landscape is not subject to analysis or correction; it's not subtle, restrained or refined. It's factual in unpleasant ways and hazardous in the elements of nature. It has character — and also demands it from the animals and humans that occupy it. And thus have evolved crocs, sharks, snakes, spiders, echidnas, kangaroos, koalas and other bizarre species of nature. It's the same with the humans. Like the land, the Aussie brand is raw, untamed and dangerous. It has roots in a convict past — and the insubordinate nature has endured and at times evolved into a new kind of animal. The humour is often sarcasm, and combined with the sun, has led to some pretty thick skin. It inspires nicknames like Bazza, Fanga, Smithy, Jonesy, Nugget and Bluey. I've heard of 'Fuckface', 'Cockhead' and my little brother's mate, 'Lettuce', so named because he sits on the side, looks good, but has no substance. Character feeds itself — and in Australia, it is everywhere.

Australia is very isolated. Because there is no other electricity of note for a couple of thousand kilometres in every direction, from space Perth looks like a star. I tell you what else is interesting, since I'm on the subject of animals and Australia. It has to do with the evolution of species. On continents, mammals tend towards gigantism and reptiles tend towards dwarfism. On islands it's the opposite; hence Australia's crocodiles, snakes and lizards. As far as humans go, especially surfers, the Australian surfer has evolved into quite an animal as well. Maybe it's the isolation.

To say that Australia is not exposed to other cultures is not true. We live in a multi-cultural society, born from European settlers. There is no such thing as an Australian restaurant, but there are Thai, Chinese, Japanese and Indian. However, there is one thing that is Australian — and it's the land, occupied by Aborigines, English convicts, European job seekers and Asian opportunity seekers. There's a bit of that in us all, either in our blood, our hearts, or our bellies.

As it is a country of beachgoers, crowds and localism can become an issue. It can get pretty nasty. Surfing doesn't operate on rules, but through common respect and etiquette. It's administered by the forefathers, then beaten into the grommets, who in turn beat it into the tourists, while the forefathers look on proudly or regretfully at the cycle of surf culture. Growing crowds and aggression in Australia have led to discussions about the possibility of implementing rules. But we all know there are no rules with Mother Nature — and she administers our day-to-day activities with more authority than a political party could ever achieve. The waves usually decide our direction.

Whether he competes, is learning, or is somewhere in between, there is a bit of the animal in the Australian surfer — unrestrained and unrefined like the land.

## LAP OF TASSIE

The change was sudden. Rain bucketed down from all angles, dropping like nails from the newly formed black sky. Massive winds whipped up white horses that rode straight over us, trampling the line-up and ending our surf with an evil wrath. Just ten minutes earlier, the hot sun had been lighting up the slightly chilled air, turning whatever our steamers couldn't cover into a burnt red through the cloudless sky.

'Don't worry, cobbers.' Our host Chris Westcott was laughing his head off. 'You're in Tasmania now, cobbers. But don't worry. If you don't like the weather, just wait a minute — it will change. It always bloody does, cobbers.'

The weather yo-yo had done its first loop and we were in the land of ocker Australians. Down under, Down Under.

It is an unfortunate fact that Tasmania has some evil connotations. Even its Dutch discoverer, Abel Tasman, named it Van Diemen's Land when he arrived in 1642. Tasmanian devils are not served well by their appearance and are aptly named. Apples are grown here, holding the knowledge of all things good and evil. I reckon the locals would laugh in the face of these apparent evils. They provide the perfect decoy to ensure that they keep one of Australia's most beautiful places to themselves. Surfers especially, who guard their waves like a secret love affair.

Being an island state, Tasmania's isolation has kept it a few years behind the rest of Australia, but at the same time, this had preserved much of its natural beauty and character. Abalone divers rule, pulling in about $50,000 on a good day, harvesting abalone to tickle the tastebuds of the Japanese elite. An abalone diving licence would cost you about nine million, in case you were wondering. Tasmania's capital, Hobart, has a population of 130,000. You can drive through the whole town without getting a stoplight.

The most forgotten evil to come out of Tasmania is the treatment of the Aborigines. When Tasmania separated from the mainland during the meltdown of the last ice age, about 10,000 years ago, the Aborigines flourished, despite being clothed in nothing more than charcoal and grease even in the coldest months. As European colonies developed, however, fighting broke out with

Aboriginal tribes. Martial law was declared in 1828, giving soldiers the right to shoot any Aborigine found on European land. Since in Aboriginal culture land can't be owned, this happened a lot. The Aborigines were driven out of Tassie and placed on the neighbouring 'civilised' and 'Christianised' Bass Strait Islands until the last full-blooded Aboriginal died in the late nineteenth century.

Driving around Tasmania looking for surf we came across plenty of Aboriginal sites. It was like walking through an isolated museum, and evoked a sense of emptiness far greater than Tasmania itself.

Since we are on the subject of evil, we may as well mention Martin Bryant. It was a pretty eerie feeling to stand on top of the hill at Port Arthur. A monument stands where thirty-five people lost their lives at the hands of that crazy man, who, unfortunately for us, was associated with surfing because of his long blond hair and a surfboard that was bolted to his roof racks. Who knows — it probably never touched the water. Maybe if it had, he wouldn't have gone on the world's biggest killing spree. After seeing such a place, it's not hard to become reflective and contemplative of human behaviour.

It was 8.25 pm and I entered the Marrawah pub on the northwest coast. After a long drive from Hobart, I walked into a stone cold reception in a quiet coastal town. As Australian as I am, I felt like a Chinese boat person because of the unwelcoming glances I received. Stacked up against the town's best flannelette shirts, ugh boots and well-groomed mullets, our latest surf gear didn't stand a chance.

'Hi,' I said nervously.

'G'day!' The lady was correcting me, not greeting me. Her local tongue shot me down in a xenophobic rage, even though I drew first. We spent the rest of the night wounded in the corner of the room, listening to the juke box pump out some of the best country and western numbers while the six locals waltzed, sipped beer and chewed on beef jerky, with or without their partners. It was Valentine's Day.

Tassie is a bit of an unknown when it comes to surfing. Though Tasmanians are surrounded by water and a lot of them make their living off the ocean, few of them ride waves. I'd talked to a lot of abalone divers who watch the swell closer than anyone, looking for a break to get out there for an easier catch. On the west coast, it doesn't happen often. 'We get a lot of swell around here,' said one local. 'But we get a lot of wind. Apparently it's one of the best places in the world to wind surf.'

We were on a camping trip and we spent most nights huddled around the campfire, drinking Boag's draught and toasting marshmallows, finally coming to rest on a mattress of boardbags with a sleeping bag for warmth. My anticipation of waves kept me awake all night and I stuck my ear to the edge of the tent like it was a giant seashell, hoping for the sweet sounds of swell.

We found it at the southernmost point of Australia, accessible only by a two-hour walk or by boat. We took the latter, though I hear this walk is famous, made sweet by the backdrop of the Southern Ocean and miles of pristine beaches. The paths are probably as busy as the roads — and they were both busy with animals. On the roads, although vehicles were sparse, there was a lot of road kill. Massive wombats walked freely across the road, snakes sunbaked on the hot tar and echidnas flirted with a tyre-flattened destiny.

Later, sitting in Hobart airport, I took some time to reflect. It's not a busy airport, but people busied themselves: leaving or returning to a place of their choice seems to add an element of excitement to airports. It's a good place to people watch, to get some quiet time and think. Sometimes I look around, but usually I'm just staring blankly.

Outside, a huge band of black cloud interrupted my train of thought with a sense of déjà vu. The change would be sudden. Rain would bucket down from all angles.

My plane was due to take off in fifteen minutes. Just in time. I looked back at Chris and pointed to the winds of change. I indicated the storm, and with my newfound Aussie twang commented, 'Don't worry, cobber — it will clear up in an hour or so.'

'Yeah, it'll probably be pumping down the coast again, too,' he replied with a confident grin. Bastards! I guess not everything in Tasmania is evil after all.

## MILLION DOLLAR BABY

Surfing is not what it used to be. Its evolution has come full circle, from the sport of kings in Hawaii, to the society outcasts, to a multi-million dollar business today.

When the Duke showed Isabel Letham into a wave at Freshwater Beach back in 1915, he had no idea that Australia would soon become the authority on surf performance, culture, fashion and industry. Islands are perfectly suited for surfing and since Australia is the biggest island in the world, the progression seemed natural. The biggest three surf companies — Billabong, Rip Curl and Quiksilver — are all Australian born. Their fashions are worn by everyone from grommets to business tycoons, from Bondi to Uluru (Ayers Rock), from LA to London.

Even former prime minister Bob Hawke walked along the beach with two-time world champ Tommy Carroll, in a pair of Quiksilver boardies and a new board when he was campaigning for office.

Back at Bondi, an eleven-year-old kid was doing his thing. He hasn't seen Tassie, Snapper or West Oz yet, but has seen pictures in the magazines. It was the weekend and his mum had dropped him and his best mate down there for an early surf. They wanted to hit it before the crowds. They always laughed at the drunken people eating doner kebabs outside the Bondi Hotel and played tricks on the ones asleep on the beach, placing bluebottles in their hair. They have dreams of being professional, of being able to surf every day of their lives, travelling the world and seeing new places — the evolution and infusement of the Australian 'walkabout'. Together they made false promises of an alcohol-free life. They touched their toes twice, put their leg ropes on and hit the water. The sun was starting to show, clocking on as the streetlights clocked off.

Within minutes, one of them was cutting through the crowd on a little right-hander, finishing off with a little air in the shorey. He had sponsors' stickers all over his board and would be called a child prodigy in any other part of the world. In America, he would already be earning more money than you or me. But in Australia, he was just one of the two million people that surf. Maybe one day he can be like his hero, Mick Fanning, but right now, he is just in the moment — looking for his own true blue.

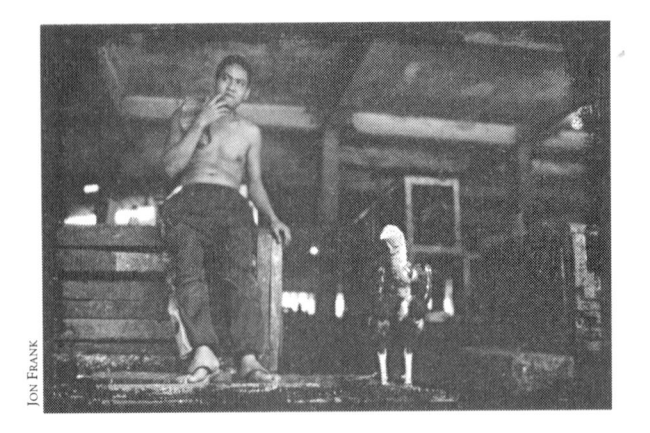

# 17,508
## INDONESIA

One thousand years ago, a whole village of Balinese people threw themselves off the cliffs of Uluwatu to escape the invading Japanese. They fell to their deaths at a place where they believed the spirits dwelled, next to a majestical cave and adjacent to the rhythm of one of the most perfect waves in the world. Over 900 years later, and escaping for different reasons, surfers have been doing the same — throwing themselves over the cliffs to experience this sacred shrine, the hallowed of all that is hollow. Over the years, travellers have come to love Bali; enjoying the richness of its Hindu culture, prospering from the personality of its people and becoming wealthy in the currency of its waves. Bali's discovery by surfers in 1971 was the prelude to surfing's equivalent of the Gold Rush, as wave riders started to unearth one of the world's best surfing destinations — Indonesia. When you think about it, it really does make sense. Indonesia is on and around the equator, so the water and weather are toasty. It's perfectly distanced from the big storms of the world's most active ocean, so the angry swells become lined up and orderly by the time they arrive. Indonesia is made up of 17,508 islands just waiting for waves to peel past an archipelago of over 5000 kilometres of coastline. It didn't take long for people to realise Indo's potential, and its diversity has inspired a pilgrimage that even malaria, pirates, earthquakes and bombs can't halt.

## BALI

Back in 1970, a fifteen-year-old school kid named Steve Cooney surfed the first wave at Uluwatu. This moment was captured by Alby Falzon and glorified in his epic film *Morning of the Earth*. When they arrived at Uluwatu along a potholed track, monkeys watched from the barren cliff with only the salt air for company and the nearby villagers went about their business of drying their fish and harvesting their rice. Now, there is a hotel on these cliffs, and at any one time, hundreds of luxury cars can be found driving along the now paved road, delivering a horde of visitors who are all eager to feel what Steve first experienced — with everything from massages to T-shirts to fill the gaps of their holiday experience.

It is a fact that nobody smiles like the Balinese. Everyone who has been there has a personal story of their friendliness — how someone on the beach they met ten years earlier remembered their name; how the Balinese laugh and smile and dance and sing; of their at times cheeky nature. But as they say in Uluwatu, 'Better cheeky than cranky'. As far as way of life goes, the Balinese have taught us more than we've taught them.

It is for these reasons and more that one of the world's best surf photographers, Jason Childs, has made Bali his home.

'I first visited Bali in 1989,' said Jason. 'I was a wide-eyed Aussie surfer/snapper on my first overseas trip. It amazed me. The people, the smells, the temples, the culture, the colours and the surf blew me away, and a seed was sown in my heart and soul.'

After his first trip, Jason's life changed.

'I can't claim that it was my great idea,' he admitted, 'but in October 1994 my wife was offered a job in the surf industry in Bali and I came along for the ride. Not long after, I realised what a great opportunity it was and that I should have thought of it myself.

'We have a great lifestyle. We work hard but our free time is our own. This allows me to indulge my three passions: family, photography and surfing. I don't mow lawns, iron shirts or wash too many dishes these days. We aren't trapped in the materialistic world of the West. Instead, I'm able to devote some of my free time to helping foundations and charities that have been set up in Indonesia by friends. These foundations help and support many poor people in this country.'

If there was ever a rupture to this peaceful way of life, it was on 12 October 2002, when the deadliest terrorist attack in Indonesian history killed 202 people, 164 of whom were foreigners. It shook the ground in more ways than one; before that, Bali had been seen as a safe haven. 'We were holidaying in Australia when the 2002 bombings happened and in many ways we were spared the pain that our friends endured. It was hard to believe that this could happen in paradise.' Yet it wasn't over. 'In 2005, the bombings at the fish cafes in Jimbaran Bay happened 200 metres from our house. As soon as we heard the explosions we ran to the beach to help. That night I saw things that I never want to see again. Because of this, I constantly remember how precious life is and that I need to live life to the fullest. Cherish the good times, get over the bad times; don't regret anything and remember how fortunate we are to have our love and our health.'

The terrorist attacks affected the Balinese people the most. Their biggest industry — more or less their only industry — was tourism. Suddenly, shops were empty, flights were empty — and people's pockets were empty. The industry they had come to rely on had deserted them, but not totally.

'The Australian government continues to issue travel warnings, but surfers seem undeterred and continue to arrive in droves on the Island of the Gods. I think that the travel warnings have really only affected families or first-time visitors to Bali. Locals, visiting surfers and others are still partying as hard. Bali continues to bounce back — the streets and hotels are buzzing again,' explained Jason.

It was surfers who first discovered Bali as a travel destination and inspired others to visit her shores for more than just the surf. Now, post bombings, different kinds of people are coming.

'There are fewer first-time Aussies and families, but Asian travellers are now discovering Bali as well as the new super-rich Russians. More surfers than ever are visiting Bali, that's for sure.

'There is nowhere else in the world like Bali. It caters to every type of tourist. The warmth of the people, the food, the weather, the culture, the cold beer and the pumping surf make it the best place in the world for a holiday on any budget.'

Jason and his wife Lisa have no immediate plans to go anywhere. Though they go back to Melbourne nearly every Christmas, they no longer consider it home.

'My wife and I love Bali. This is our home. We love Indonesia and the people. Indonesia has been very good to us. It's an amazing place to live, to be a photographer and a surfer.'

Soon after Bali was first surfed, the question was being asked: If Bali is this good, surely in the thousands of islands that make up Indonesia, there is another place that is even better? It didn't take long for people to do the hard yards to find out. Enter Peter Troy.

## SHRINKING HEADS AND CANNIBALISM

It was the hippies and the surfers who first visited most of Indonesia, and there was one of their number who took the exploration a little further: Peter Troy, surfing's equivalent of Forrest Gump. He was the first to ride a shortboard in Australia, the man who started the oldest surfing event at Bells Beach. He hitchhiked around the world in the sixties, through the Arctic Circle, across the Sahara and to Mount Everest. He introduced surfing to Brazil. And just when you might have expected him to keep his thumb in his pocket, he came up with the idea of riding a motorbike from Bells to Bali.

I met Peter in 2002 when I featured him in my last book, *Surfers*. During my research, we met at his home on the Sunshine Coast and talked about his experiences in Indonesia.

'In 1970, '71 and '72, the first guys were going to Indo. I was in that vanguard when I first surfed at Uluwatu; I got a surfboard embedded in my back and nearly lost my life there. Then I thought I could sail an Indonesian boat back to Australia, but the boat sank, so I was left sitting in Indo wondering what to do next. I could have gone over and maybe discovered G-Land, but in actual fact I was going the other way. I did end up in Timor but didn't really know there was surf there. I got on a yacht and went north around

Timor and ended up in Darwin, so I didn't see the surf. Of course, this is just the way the world is — you're not going to see those things all the time.

'Then my vision was of travelling through the whole of Southeast Asia on my own motorbike. When I came back to Australia in 1974, I decided that I was going to ride to Nepal. The plan was that my girlfriend and I were going to ride a 200cc motorbike to Darwin, go over to Timor, go right up through Indo to Thailand, take a plane to Nepal, then travel round Nepal and down through India. Then I was going to live in the Seychelle Islands for the rest of my life.

'But then Cyclone Tracy hit Darwin in December 1974 and the city was closed, so we couldn't ride our motorbikes there. Instead, we got on a cruise boat with the bikes and went on a *Women's Weekly* cruise with sixty, seventy and eighty year olds up to Hong Kong. The ship stopped in Bali where they put our motorbikes on a life raft, and dropped us over the side without passing any immigration or customs. So, we revved up the motorbikes and started driving. Eight months later, after riding the motorbikes through jungles, up mountains, and carrying them up the sides of cargo boats, my girlfriend and I discovered Nias. We had actually driven through the jungles of Sumatra along the west coast, and had looked down on the Mentawai. We knew there would be waves there, but there was no way we could ever get out there. So we missed all of that. But then again we were actually the first surfers to get to Nias.'

Peter later read a strange story about this time that quite unnerved him. It had been written by a guy who had been with him in Nias when they discovered it.

'The story, which is incredible, was told by Kevin Lovett, who was asked by SBS to go back and research it for a documentary. He'd already lived in Indonesia for many years so his Bahasa Indonesian was good. When he went back to where we had been in Nias, he looked up all the kids and people who had looked after him, and he talked to the man who, as a ten year old, brought our food to us. He was now thirty-two years old and had been influenced by all the surfers who'd come to Nias and now ran a shop.

'He told us that they thought we'd come from another planet and that when we were sitting on our surfboards, we were actually catching fish and taking away their food. They had no idea that we were surfing! Because they were scared that we were taking their food, they went to consult their witch doctor. He actually put potions into the food that was being taken out to us at the camp — so they were slowly poisoning us. We were to be sacrificed on the point, where there were already skulls from other tribes.

'Kevin's story, which was published in *Surfers Journal*, made incredible reading because, when they went back a second time, his girlfriend became extremely ill and nearly died. Also, one of the three of us who had first been there lost his life a few months later, in Afghanistan. I didn't stay there long enough for the poison to work on me. For some reason I was on the road again on my motorbike.

'It's quite frightening in a way because it shows the innocence that you travel with throughout the world. It's the same everywhere. It doesn't matter if you're in the jungles of the Amazon or on the beaches of Indonesia. Your life can end just like that. You might think it's a great adventure to use a blow dart to shoot a monkey or look at shrunken human heads. You might see them in the hut that you're living in, and think, "Oh well, there are five shrunken heads," but you don't imagine that you might become one of them. You don't realise that you might be doing something wrong according to their culture that might make them decide to take your life. This is really a realisation for all of us who surf, whether we're just going to one of the islands in the Seychelles or to the Andaman Islands. We walk in there as very naive travellers. We could accidentally end up in a jail in Bangkok or Turkey for the rest of our lives. We could be up in the north of Sumatra and go to a place where the Muslims don't want you. Life's very cheap.'

## BOMBS, TSUNAMIS, VOLCANOES AND BEDLAM IN THE BLOOD

Indonesia is at the centre of an enormous push to revive tourism, resulting in surfers arriving en masse — and profiting in some way — from the perfect waves. Still, throughout the country, there is poverty and corruption — the result of bombs going off, volcanoes exploding, earthquakes, tsunamis and bedlam in the blood. The corruption was obvious on our drive to Uluwatu, when we bribed the policeman to ignore our lack of an international driving licence. We also saw it on the streets and in the outer islands of Sumatra. You don't have to look far — the realities of Indonesia will always find you. Unfortunately, the Indonesians are not equipped to handle all these disasters, but they have to live with them on a daily basis. One such bedfellow is malaria — or what they call the 'hot/cold fever'.

Malaria has killed more people in the history of the world than anything else — and the problem is getting worse. In 2008, malaria will strike half a billion people, mostly Africans, but it is an epidemic encompassing 106 developing nations. Indonesians suffer immensely from the disease and in the outer islands the people can't afford to spray

DDT, cut wetlands, or wrap their children in mosquito nets. Robert Gwadz, who has studied malaria at the National Institute of Health near Washington DC for almost thirty-five years, wrote in an article in *National Geographic*, 'In its ability to adapt and survive, the malaria parasite is a genius. It's smarter than we are.'

But not everyone can accept that.

Dr Dave Jenkins, a surfer/doctor from Australia, has enlisted the support of the people who profit from these islands to help the locals with medical aid. Thus was born Surfaid — 'a non-profit humanitarian aid organisation to improve the health of people living in isolated regions connected to us through surfing.'

'It can be a hard place to live,' said Albert Taylor, a surf charter boat skipper who lives in Sumatra. 'Malaria is a huge problem — and then there's the constant threat of earthquakes.'

On 26 December 2004 an undersea earthquake triggered a series of tsunamis which, with waves up to thirty metres high, hit the west coast of Sumatra, killing more than 225,000 people. It was one of the deadliest natural disasters in history. With a magnitude of between 9.1 and 9.3 on the Richter scale, it was the second largest earthquake ever recorded. It caused the entire planet to vibrate by as much as a centimetre and triggered other earthquakes as far away as Alaska. Seven billion US dollars were given by countries around the world in aid and, while the island is starting to recover, fear is still ever present.

'I lived in Padang from 1996 to 2006 until earthquakes drove me out of there,' Albert told me. 'Experts are saying there will be plenty more. I've moved my family further above sea level in case another tsunami comes. The last one was pretty devastating. The whole configuration of the ocean bed and the reefs changed. It was pretty radical!'

This was just another natural disaster in a very turbulent area. In 1883, a bomb went off. It was heard as far away as Perth and Mauritius and was recognised as the loudest noise recorded in modern history. It was equivalent to 200 megatonnes of TNT, or about 13,000 times more powerful than the atomic bomb that devastated Hiroshima in 1945. Around 36,417 people — the official toll — were killed from the blast and the resulting tsunamis. It was the most powerful volcanic eruption ever: its name was Krakatoa.

In October 2002 another bomb went off. But this was a new kind of bomb that Indonesians were not used to. It happened on a small peaceful Hindu island in the middle of a Muslim archipelago. In the tourist district of Kuta, the deadliest act of terrorism in the history of Indonesia killed more than 200 people.

'Many tourists coming back to Bali,' said Katut, who owns a store selling T-shirts, carvings and jewellery. 'We don't want problem. We just want everyone to be happy.'

## ANWAR STAR

At first I was disappointed to learn that the pronunciation of One Anwar's first name was actually 'Oni'. It should be the name of a president or philosopher, or at least a self-named rapper or pimp wearing the fake fur of an endangered animal. But it's not. The name is owned and operated by a thirteen-year-old grommet from Lakey Peak on the island of Sumbawa. However, after a day or two of hanging out with him, it becomes clear that fame will come — and in his own creative way. Like many Indonesian grommets, he was exposed to travelling surfers and learned how to surf on their broken boards on slapping reef-covered shorebreaks. Before long, his feet turned to leather, his blood turned to salt, and he became one of the best surfers of Lakey Peak. He is fast, both on his board and with his mouth. 'I start surf when I was maybe seven. Yeah, and I just try every day since. I love it. Now it's my life.'

One is your typical cheeky Indo grom. When he's not cracking jokes, he's thinking about the next one. Due to his time in the surf, his skin is darker than most Indonesians. And he surfs so much that there isn't the time to eat enough nasi gorengs to lend bulk to his growing frame.

One recently received an invitation to go to Bali. His sponsor offered to pay him to go to school, learn English, and have the opportunity to improve as a surfer. I meet One during a training camp we had organised for young stars, which included our best under-eighteen surfers from Australia, New Zealand and Indonesia. One was the youngest of the group, but I soon realised he had something special. The Indonesian team manager, Yuda, did also. One lives with Yuda, his sponsor, who is doing a great job of helping him balance his life between the responsibilities of homework and the opportunities of professional surfing. One thanks Yuda not only by winning every event in his age division but also by winning open events, against some of his more famous peers like Rizal Tanjung. His is a name we should all write down.

The first day of the training camp, Yuda had to call One's school and tell them he was ill in order to give him the opportunity to train with myself and the other kids. 'I only ever take him out of school if it's a big competition, or the surf is pumping,' said Yuda, who is little more than a grommet himself.

'Bali is the place to be to have a good life. If you came to Bali twenty-five years ago there was nothing here, just some coconut trees. Now we have good communication, internet, but also some pollution and bad people coming. Bali has changed a lot. But if these kids can surf for a job, that will be very good, so we try to make them learn the good life.'

'School's okay,' admitted One, as we headed towards Canguu for our first surf. 'We learn Indonesian language and English, but today was maths, so I want to surf instead!'

And so we did. It was three to four feet and one of the best performance waves was just starting to show the effects of the resident tradewinds chopping its face. He may only be young, but One has an incredible talent. He was doing air reverses and stalling for barrels, even hitting a lip three times his height.

'So many surfers are now here. Every day I can surf with somebody who surfs amazing. People from Bali like Petit and Mega, but also people on the WCT are coming to Bali all the time. I love surfing with them and learning and I hope one day to be a pro like them,' One told me.

He is well on his way. If he can do what he did in Bali with a steamer on, in cold water and in an alien place, he could be the best Indonesian surfer to date. All signs point in that direction. But there is also another thing holding him back — why would you want to leave the warm perfection of Bali?

Mega is a little older than One, and is beginning to ask himself those same questions. He also rides for Rip Curl and has started to do Search trips with the likes of Mick Fanning and Taylor Knox, which is helping him to improve. He surfs all day, every day, in perfect waves, chases girls when the sun falls orange over the horizon, then does it all over again. It's a good life — but it didn't start that way.

'I started surfing when I was seven. My uncle used to make me play sports. I played soccer and badminton. Then one day I tried to surf. I have surfed every day since.'

We stopped in at his house one day on our way to Uluwatu. It's on the main road just before you get to the turn-off for Bingin. Incense burned amongst flowers, rice and water — an expression of their Hindu beliefs. His mum smiled in welcome; she was proud of the life her son had created. He had clothes on his back, did something he loved and enjoyed his life. For that, she gave extra thanks to Ganesha, the elephant-headed supreme being. I'm actually not sure if that's correct. Maybe it was to Garuda, who communicates messages between the heavens and man. In any case, she was proud of her son.

Mega dedicates a lot of time to walking to the surf from his home. 'It took me maybe one hour every day to walk to Bingin to learn surfing. I would try to borrow a board and start to learn. People would break boards there, so I could ride half a board, or some days I would get lucky and people would let me borrow a whole one.'

I talked to Mega just after he placed third in the Dompu Open at Lakey Peak where he won the equivalent of US$1000 in rupiah. The kid is starting to make money not only for himself, but for his family. He can afford a phone, a car and a life his parents could only watch on Western TV shows, if they could even afford a TV.

'Yeah, we have many contests now. The Indonesian circuit is good. First place is twenty million rupiah, so it's good.' That's over US$2000. 'And there are more and more events every year.'

Mega is leading the way for One and a host of other Indonesian kids. Their Hindu upbringing and peaceful nature doesn't lend itself very well to the rigours of tough competition on the world scale;

however, that doesn't matter, because the world is coming to them. They can stay in Bali, do trips to the outer islands, make money from the domestic circuit and stay home, living a healthy lifestyle near the ocean. Pretty good for a culture that less than forty years ago thought the ocean was a place of evil spirits.

## G-LAND

There was a constant commotion in the camp at Grajagan (G-land), stirred up by everyone from young pros to seasoned sea-dogs who have spent enough time in Indonesia to warrant a Javanese passport and an immunity to malaria. Off slip the winter wax jobs and the thought of steamers. That's the first act of foreplay. Rockers and bottom curves are carefully caressed, leg ropes slip through pin tails; wax, sunscreen, mozzie nets and booties are found.

I went to G-land a few years ago with Luke Egan, who won the Quiksilver Pro in '97. 'It's my seventh time here,' he said. Luke spoke with a soft monotone that doesn't need pitch, as his conversation always has enough range. 'For one spot, it can change so much. I've never surfed it the same twice. There are so many different sections to it — Kongs, Money Trees, Speedies.' His love for this wave is reflected in his ability to surf it. He drew pictures with his hands of waves barrelling over different sections. If there is a wave for Luke Egan, G-land is it.

I bumped into Matt Archibold while I was there, who was with the O'Neill team from America. Tom Curren once rated him as one of the most naturally talented surfers in the world and I've always had a fascination for his surfing. 'Hi, I'm Matt,' I said, introducing myself.

'So am I,' he replied. Archie was a soulman, inked in coolness. While the rest of the team watched the footage of the day, Archie sat with his back to the monitor, blowing cigarette smoke at the full moon. It was the only time I have ever considered cigarette smoking cool.

'This place is so crazy for rats,' said Tommy Reyes, whose chocolate stash had been raided by vermin. The jungle has many surprises. It's a place where people talk about booties, dream of perfect barrels, envision tigers, eat nasi goreng and fart with little confidence. Stories abound of rats the size of dogs, wild cats the size of bears, mosquitoes like bats and bats like 747s. Meanwhile, Krakatoa sits menacingly to the west. People say it's ready to go off again. They also predict another tidal wave like the one that left Richard Marsh and Richie Lovett in a tree in the middle of the night, bruised, battered and broken, contemplating the fragility of where the jungle meets the sea. Who knows? There have been more tidal waves since that one in '94 and a brown, dinged-up, broken board hangs in Bobby's camp as a silent reminder. It had never been ridden.

One day a young kid named Jon Jon Florence, who was eleven at the time, came running into the dining area and told his worried mum about the green, ribbon-shaped snake they had just been playing with. It turns out the snake was a green mamba and could have killed them within minutes. 'In the rain, snakes are always coming,' said Puma, the local wiseman, who had been working in the camp since its inception. I asked him what other animals he had seen in the camp.

'I have seen the tiger once in '93,' he recalled. 'But I don't think they are around here anymore. Maybe three black cats.' He flashed a wary grin through his yellow teeth. 'Also leopards. There are many leopards here.' The local camp workers enjoy the lifestyle there, a credit to the camp's owner, Bobby, who pays them more than he has to.

Not as many people come to G-land as they used to. Why would you come to one wave, when you can do a boat trip in the Mentawais, or chase a variety of waves in Bali or the Sumbawa region? But that doesn't influence Louie. 'I'll be back,' he said. 'I always come back.'

## LOVE BOAT CAPTAIN

There are many oceans. Sometimes the ocean is as calm as a giant pond, flat and reflective like a great mirror. Sometimes the remnants of a far away storm send rhythmic lines through a calm surface, hypnotic in their order. There's an ocean that rises into moving mountains, like the Andes liquefying and moving across the Pacific with menace on the mind. Also, the sky tends to vary a lot more over water and is rarely completely cloudless. Water to the sky is like paint to an artist. Sometimes the clouds look like cotton wool, sometimes like fluffy pillows. If you stare at them long enough, you can turn them into shapes and objects. There are white ones, grey ones, black ones; the ocean and the sky are in constant communication. Some clouds give off colour, some give off rain — and some give off lightning and thunder. This is a common occurrence around the equator, which is so far away from the poles that it lacks electricity in the atmosphere, so thunderstorms are nature's way of electrifying the air. Sometimes the storms are on the horizon; sometimes you can hear them without seeing them. And sometimes you can hear them and see them at the same time.

As a skipper in the Mentawai Islands, Albert Taylor has seen it all. He has spent the better part of his life sleeping with the ocean beneath him, the stars above him and the nautical maps beside him. He's been around the elements for so long that they are now a part of him. Bert skippers the *Indies Trader 2*, which is owned by Rip Curl's founder, Doug Warbrick, and current CEO, Francois Payot. It was on this boat that I got to know Bert.

'I grew up in Warilla, in the Barrack Point area, south of Wollongong,' Albert, who has a way of drawing you into the conversation, told us. 'I started going to Bali in the early eighties as an eighteen-year-old. In '82 I survived by fishing with the Kuta reef locals. They used to laugh at me because I used a fishing rod. In August 1983, I met Brett Haysom and I organised two trips to G-land on the beautiful gaff-rigged ketch *Ann Judith 2* — an ex-World War II mine-sweeping vessel which Brett had salvaged in Perth. After the two trips Brett offered me a full-time job on the vessel from April till November.

'We travelled to G-land, Desert Point and the Scar Reef regions for the next five years. Deserts, Lombok and Sumbawa were unreal. We weren't the first there, but what an experience. We would rarely see another soul, let alone another charter boat. Brett was the first real professional surf charter pioneer. He is a professional top-shelf maritime soul.

'In '88 I started working full-time; I sailed east to Nusatengara, Sumba, Sawu and Timor until '91. It was unreal; there were no crowds, just opportunity. In 1991, Mark Coleman and I completed building the *Nusa Dewata* and sailed it to Timor. During the building of the *Dewata* I had been introduced to Martin Daly and later found myself working for him in the Mentawais in August of '94. I sailed 90 per cent of the journey from Sumatra to the Tuamotos.'

Albert has a saying: 'Just square it away and put it to bed.' Whether he was giving orders to his deckhands pulling up anchor or advising us about the ladies, he would insist that a job is not done until you put it to bed. 'First you have to square it away,' said Bert. 'But it's not done until you put it to bed.'

From then on, we squared away surfs and put beers to bed. 'Albert, just going to square away my boards,' Mick Fanning would say.

'Roger that, Mick, just don't forget to put them to bed by tying them up. We're moving soon.' We loved it. We would often join Albert in his quarters, looking at his maps and talking with him about life on the ocean. The region has changed a lot since it first exploded in the mid-nineties. There are now over forty charter boats up there — and most of the surfing photos and footage you see has been shot in this region.

'Life up here now is very different. Although there are lots of charter boats, the general attitude is pretty good as the current skippers all work pretty well together — except for Bucket.' I guess there's always one. Maybe Bucket, whoever he is, hasn't yet learned to square things away AND put them to bed?

'The number of visitors to the islands has risen along with diesel prices, but on most occasions you still enjoy unreal, uncrowded waves. You've just got to travel a little and utilise a bit of local knowledge, to surf uncrowded perfect waves,' Bert explained.

'Some spots have risen six feet out of the water since the tsunami, so the search has been rejuvenated for the hidden gems that lie around the corner. This is unreal, because it gives you a second wind of enthusiasm.'

Bert has lived here for a while now, skippering three kids and starting a coffee plantation business on the side, but his life clearly revolves around the ocean.

'I used to dream about Sumatra and tigers when I was eight. Now I'm married to one,' he laughs. 'My Sumatran wife is splendid and I've got a good life here with my three great kids. I miss them when I'm working the boats, but ending up as one of the luckiest surfers on the planet has helped to balance me. It makes for a pretty happy smile on your face at the end of the day. During that evolution, I've been pretty blessed with great times, friends, adventures and the odd wave.'

He's also grown close to the culture and way of life of this developing country.

'The Mentawai people are very different. There are two types: the beach dwellers, who are a mixture of real locals and transmigrants, and the real Mentawai forest dwellers. I have never really got to know them as I have always been trying to keep the boat afloat. I will say that there has been a lot of very quick change here, with some positives and some negatives. When we used to surf back in the day, a local in a canoe would not even look at you. By 2007, they were telling me where I could and couldn't anchor the boat. However, those kind of people are in the minority and most of the locals are really hospitable people.

'The worst part of my life here is when I'm in the dinghy and you blokes are surfing. But I've had my turn and sharing many good waves with a lot of great friends is a good way to spend your life — surfing, fishing, Bintang [the beer in Bali], sunsets …

'The main negative point is being in the surf and seeing, one — people can't wait their turn in the line-up; and two — the instant local. But after a couple of years of doing the job, the good points well outnumber the bad points.'

'What about the future?' I asked. Bert looked over the front deck, past the empty Bintangs, the stickered surfboards and camera equipment, towards the ocean that was displaying its many moods, as if it still hadn't decided what to do. Beyond the starboard side, palm trees danced in the wind and afternoon fires sent up smoke to keep the malaria mosquitoes at bay. Little village boys became silhouettes as they paddled their unsold carvings back to their homes, and the odd flying fish had a quick look before diving back into the ocean. Bert thought about the question and put the answer to bed. 'The future. Mmm … bad eyes, earthquakes, some squabbling over Mother Nature — and a lot of perfect waves.'

INDONESIA

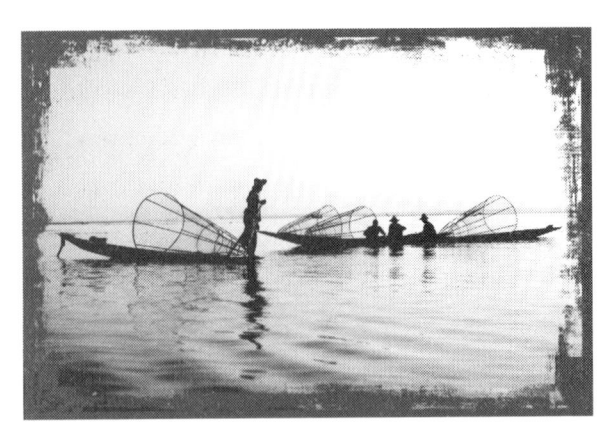

# BEYOND CLOUD NINE
## PHILIPPINES

'The low tropical pressure system is predicted to intensify into a typhoon.' Scott Countryman was delivering the best possible welcome speech as we boarded his impressive vessel, the *King of Sports*. 'What normally happens with these typhoons in the Philippines is they tend to fizzle out and move towards us, not producing much swell. But this one looks perfect. It's supposed to get a lot stronger, move out to sea — and sit here.' His finger jabbed a spot on his nautical map 500 miles east of the Philippines, the world's second-largest archipelago. His finger danced on the map in circles, mimicking the brewing storm and crinkling the paper in a violent display of what was about to occur. We were on one of 7017 (mainly undiscovered) islands that make up the Philippines — and we were about to enter the largely uncharted waters.

Australians Andy King, Jay Thomson and young superstar Brent Dorrington crowded around the map, as if pulled in by the spinning storm. It was their first time to the Philippines — and a huge swell was about to wash away any preconceived notions about a place often referred to as 'the Fickle-pines'. With this storm, we would be able to fulfil our goal; not only would we find waves, but we would get some too. Tiny islands were all around us, wrapped generously by green palm trees and blue swell. Scott turned from the weather fax to his nautical maps to show where we'd be surfing. He had written 'potential spot' twenty-six times. The imagery was exciting: countless islands, some small and some big, dotted the equatorial blue. Some of the islands in the Philippines are surrounded by shallow reefs which can drop away suddenly to a dark and dangerous 10,000 feet, making this part of the world, according to Scott, 'the most dangerous waters in the world'. But it hasn't deterred him. While most of the area's inhabitants hide from typhoons, Scott chases them.

'Saipan is the worst place for typhoons,' he explained. 'Basically, there are mini typhoons and super typhoons. I've seen typhoons with 287 mph winds. Cars roll away like tumbleweed and you see rusty iron ripped off roofs, fly through the air and stick into palm trees. I was in one once. It was a super typhoon and it was smashing us. Then all of a sudden, we were in the eye of the storm. It was at night and you could see the moon. Everything went still — then bang! The typhoon's tail got us bad.'

After a first afternoon of surfing at a nice left-hander, the elements turned nasty. Within two hours, half of our passengers had doubled over with seasickness. The *King of Sports* hit the open ocean and rocked over the bumpy swells before falling into dark twenty-foot troughs. The typhoon was coming — the cracking and squeaking of the boat said so. After a torrid night, everyone was lying in a different spot to the one they'd fallen asleep in, but by sunrise tranquillity had returned. While the others slept it off, Scott and I seized the opportunity to investigate some potential waves and to pay our respects to the villagers.

We parked the boat in the reedy shallows and knocked on the door of the village chief, while thirty or forty villagers gathered around us. Scott introduced me, explained what we were doing there and introduced the possibility of others coming once they saw the photos of his beautiful island.

'Please, be my guests,' the chief replied in quite good English, asking, 'Maybe just a small donation to help with water for the village?'

Some things in Asia never change. And in a tiny little village, the villagers are more than happy to continue the only philosophy that's ever worked for them: live day to day with whatever presents itself. Back in the whaler, Scott informed us about the island as we sped along its shores.

It may be one of 7017, but each island seems to have 7017 unique traits. New species are being discovered in the hills every day. Most waters are virginal. Every corner we went around had another wave yet to be named and yet to be surfed. As we sailed on, the open ocean swell was huge and was backdropped by 2000-foot high vertical mountains, jagged like broken glass. It was like the land of the giants. It was also riddled with history. The US Army had built a lighthouse here so that they could watch for the Japanese Navy during World War II. This was also the island that Ferdinand Magellan landed on in 1521 when he became the first man to circumnavigate the world (he was later killed on an island in Cebu by the locals).

Even though the Americans left here sixty years ago, there's still an army on the island today. The NPA (the New People's Army, the military wing of the Communist party) are hiding in the hills here, fighting their own guerilla campaign to overthrow the government.

Only very recently, a Brussels-based research centre declared the Philippines the most disaster-prone country on earth. It cited typhoons, earthquakes, volcanic eruptions, floods, garbage landslides and military action against Muslim insurgents as just some of the perils that locals and tourists have had to deal with. And they didn't even see the right-hander we surfed. As Scott and I watched a fifteen-footer detonate on the reef, we knew we had found something miraculous.

Before boarding the boat, our photographer, John Callahan, told us that he didn't want us surfing there. 'It's too dangerous,' he warned. 'I don't want the trip ending because there are no boards left and people need to go to hospital.' But his warnings fell on deaf ears, and we started surfing straight away. It was a lot bigger and thicker than we thought, even for a typhoon swell. Pride was tested.

The right, yet to be named, is at the edge of the northern tip of the island, and is open fully to the swell. From the six-foot-deep ledge where the wave unloaded to the 10,000-foot drop-off only a hundred feet out the back, it looked like the ocean was falling off the side of a cliff. Scott and I inspected it for around fifteen minutes. It looked impossible, like a dangerous phenomenon that should be fenced for people to sit back and watch. One set came through that had to be fifteen feet. It exploded to twice its height; it sounded like a bomb and felt like an earthquake.

Five of the eight of us on the boat paddled out, and three of us caught waves. Kingy was first up. He thrives in that sort of situation and was looking for the biggest rideable sets. Jay Thomson, who had the advantage of having his left foot forward, found some thick barrels, but to be quite honest, the biggest, or I should say squarest waves, weren't ridden — though not from lack of trying. It made me want to take back every other 'unrideable' call I'd ever made. That wave was truly a monster.

With the typhoon still in place, we set sail early the next morning in search of other virgin line-ups, joining the dots of unexplored islands. We rolled over some big clean swells that morning and everything looked in place. But by the time we crossed the strait towards Dinagat Island, the tail of the typhoon had wagged for the last time. We surfed a little right that was a good set-up, but simply too small. The fact was, we had left the swell behind. So while everyone surfed or fished, I took the boat to shore.

I met one local fisherman. He was sixty-five and only remembered taking one day off from fishing in his entire life (the day of his daughter's wedding). There are a lot of fishermen there, and they are exceptional at their job. But with everybody fishing, there are no fish left. The place is fished out. There are no rules; they use cyanide, explosives, you name it. If it's there, they'll find it, kill it, eat it or sell it — small fish, big fish, crustaceans, snails. Half the fishermen have had their hands, or half their hands, blown off because the explosives they use to get the fish have gone off too early. They will spend two or three days at a time cramped in tiny canoes, huddling in the dark and in the rain, looking for tuna or giant trevally. Sometimes typhoons come — and the fishermen don't come back. Other times they free dive, with tiny makeshift goggles made out of a bit of perspex and wood, as deep as 200 feet for minutes at a time, looking for what is no longer left at the surface. They get the bends all the time.

'They get totally fucked up,' said Scott. 'It's gnarly. They don't have any depressurising chambers or anything like that. They bury the divers in the sand up to their shoulders and wait. Some live, some die.'

The jungles here used to be alive with hard wood, mainly mahogany. But like the fish, the trees are also gone. Once the expensive hardwood ran out, the locals found that the turnaround from palm trees, which grow a lot quicker than hardwood and from which they can harvest coconuts every few months, was a much better prospect for cultivation.

In 1521, and with little bloodshed, Spain set up a colony in the Philippines that lasted 377 years. But the Spanish slowly destroyed the Filipino culture, forcing an arranged — and now divorced — marriage of Filipino, Spanish and American traditions. The US–Spanish war in the Philippines ended Spanish rule and helped to establish Filipino independence in 1898. Thus began the Americanisation of the Philippines. Shopping malls thrive and people wear shirts emblazoned with 'Team America'. It's such a weird combination of cultures. Women run around half-nude, selling their bodies; and posters of a half-naked Britney Spears are everywhere. But the Filipinos did have to censor the words in that Groove Armada song, 'I See You Baby', changing the lyric 'Shak'n that ass' to 'Shak'n that thing', because, after all, they are Catholics.

John Callahan has seen it all. He now lives in Manila and was one of the pioneers of the Philippines' surfing scene back in 1992. But he wasn't the first. It takes a certain type of eccentricity to become an explorer and that quality was certainly evident in Mike Boyum, the first man to discover the Philippines' waves. Boyum, who also discovered Grajagan, was on Siargao from January to April 1988, where he died of starvation. He had decided to fast for forty-seven days. A priest was to meet him on the forty-seventh day with food, but Boyum died a few days before. John told us that story, and he and Scott told us many more on the way to another island.

One story Scott recounted was about a mad Christian cult leader, an American who had taken up residence about a kilometre from where we were anchored.

'Ruben Ecleo was considered to be the reincarnation of Jesus Christ by about a million followers in the central and southern Philippines. When the remains of his wife were found in a rubbish bag at the bottom of a cliff in Cebu, he came to the attention of authorities. After being accused of the crime, Ecleo, who'd lived with his wife and two children in Cebu, fled to his cult headquarters on Dinagat island where thousands of sect members formed a human barricade to prevent the police from arresting him.

'After a six-month stand-off the police raided the cult mansion in an attempt to make the arrest. Cult members then opened fire on the security forces. Seventeen cult followers and one policeman died in the raid on the compound. Ecleo eventually surrendered and is now in prison awaiting trial. In prison he has also become a celebrity. He's in the local newspapers all the time.'

Eventually, the typhoon ended up leaving as quickly as it came, like a huge fire engulfing an ocean of twigs. We checked about a dozen destinations that Scott had marked on his nautical maps as 'potential spots'. But with the ocean fizzling out, they unfortunately remained just that — potential spots. Instead, we spent our time free diving and scuba diving, something that every surfer should do.

As surfers, we spend most of our time struggling to get back to the surface. Tell me the fantasy of breathing under water doesn't talk to you in capital letters. We saw some amazing things too; manta shrimp were the most bizarre. 'Don't go near it!' Scott screamed when Kingy tried to touch one. Apparently they can travel 200 metres per second and can impale you. That's faster than a .22 calibre hand cannon — and they're only the size of a hummingbird. 'Now that's fast food,' said Kingy. Someone had to say it.

With the help of the GPS, a couple of dolphins guided the vessel back to its docks in Cebu. The typhoon, the swell and the big right were well and truly behind us by then — and after setting sail into the typhoon's tail the previous week, we instead sailed head-on into the whirlwind of the Philippines' second largest city. In our travels, we had explored many islands in the Philippines. But there is so much more to discover — and it could never be done in one trip. I looked at the stars, which for the last few weeks had been burning brightly in the sky above the bow of the *King of Sports*, but their glow was stolen by the approaching city of Cebu. Above me, a buzzing satellite flew by as if late for work. Soon I would be too.

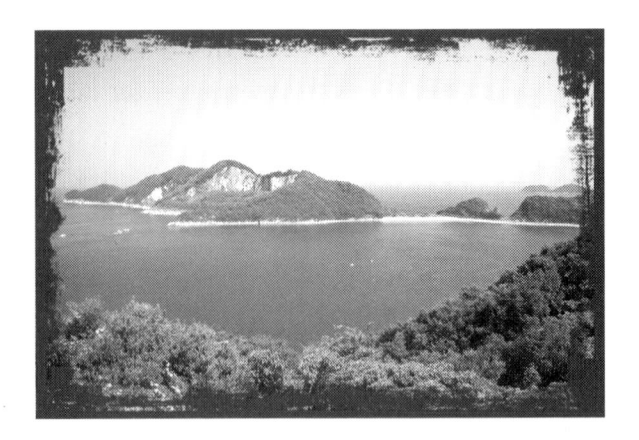

# MAYHEM AND MAMA-SAN
## JAPAN

The culture in the land of the rising sun is very strange. Search your mind for associations and you'll probably come up with some oddities: massive sumo wrestlers, ninja warriors and karate experts; swapping swords and words; bowing heads with mutual respect. That's the old Japan — and you can still find it deep in the hearts and jungles of its custodians. It's their connection to their past and to their honour — an honour so strong that some of them have become a kamikaze to defend it. Then there's the other side: ultra post-modernistic and technical futurism, where bright neon lights advertise cars and mobile phones the rest of the world won't see for years; a place where teenagers play the latest technology in massive games rooms, before retiring to a little restaurant where the owner serves eel, miso soup and green tea. Even for the hardened traveller, Japan will register higher than anywhere else as far as culture shock goes. However, somewhere between the alien ideas and the old ideals is a culture that works harmoniously.

## PLACE OF CONTRAST

On a snowboarding trip, Mick Fanning and I had cut through an illegal area, more due to our lack of control than because we were making a serious attempt at lawbreaking. We were up in Niseko celebrating Mick's world title with a snowboarding holiday — and trouble had found us swiftly. The staff chased after us into the crowded rest area where tourists, mostly Australian, were warming themselves with miso soup, chased with Asahi beer. It was there we hid. The authorities arrived in the area and scanned it with piercing eyes. But as close as we were to them, they couldn't spot us. Frustrated, they muttered something in Japanese before moving on. 'Do you know what they just said?' asked our Japanese friend. 'All these fucking round-eyes look the same.' We laughed our heads off, never having considered that we're as alien to the 128 million people who live here as they are to us.

It was then I had a realisation: to really discover Japan, we have to see it through their eyes. So — to be a little bit cheeky, let's squint and indulge in the contrast.

The characters that make up the name Japan mean 'sun-origin', which is why it is often referred to as 'the land of the rising sun'. It is a country of world champion manners; the people are elegantly dressed and super respectful. However, their national heritage also contains a tradition of massive men wrestling each other in their underpants! They live in houses and villages that are, like their people, 70 per cent smaller than those in the West. Even their cars aren't much bigger than Tonka toys; they have to be to fit through the streets and into the garages of their owners. Apart from the sumo giants, the houses are small, the trees are small and the people are small. Japan is a country that is actually 70 per cent mountainous forest. It is these forested areas that arrest the urban sprawl. Unable to spread wide, the Japanese have grown upwards, like a tree searching for sunlight in a crowded forest.

It is in the huge cities that the weirdness congregates. You can get barrelled in wave pools, snowboard synthetically under a roof in the middle of summer, then spend the night in a hotel capsule. 'The wave pool is amazing,' said Matt Wilkinson, one of Australia's best up-and-coming surfers. 'It fully barrels. It's just weird because there's a roof over your head, the water is chlorine and when you fall off, you hit cement.'

If and when you want to discover some real waves, you'll find plenty, especially in typhoon or tsunami season. There are over 3000 islands in Japan and the opportunities for waves are boundless.

## FOTO PREASE

I'm not sure of her real name; she was just 'Mama-san'. She bowed in respect every time we walked past. Years of this activity had left her 85-year-old back bent at right angles to the ground. She walked with her hands locked behind her back to offset her balance. Since her head was a long way from her centre of gravity, it took her a long time to turn around, so she only moved if it was worth taking the time to do so.

We were there for the Quiksilver Pro, the fifth event of the World Tour. Since the small village in Chiba had no hotels, we were taken in by local families who fed and housed us for the week we were there. It was at Mama-san's house that the Rip Curl team and I stayed. Upon our arrival, she bowed several times. She kept repeating the process every time our eyes met. Since she knew no English and we knew no Japanese, we communicated in backbends, head bows and hand gestures.

'Have a hug,' said Mick Fanning, immediately adopting her as his mum. He dropped into a squat to meet her at eye level and they embraced. When she finished blushing, Mama-san led us to our quarters. She motioned to her walls, which were postered with every professional surfing event that had taken place on her beach there in Japan. There were posters from Mizaka Pros in the early eighties, signed by people like Derek Ho, Martin Potter, Dave Macaulay, Richard 'Dog' Marsh, Damien Hardman, Barton Lynch, Hans Hedamen, Brad Gerlach and Tom Curren. They wrote messages like 'love your miso soup', and 'thanks for being our mum for the week'.

She had a big family. The event hadn't taken place there for a few years but it was as if we were part of her big adopted family, and she welcomed us like nephews.

Our beds were futons on the floor. It was Mick's second time in Japan, but he was still culture shocked. We left our bags on the ground and joined Mama-san for dinner. 'This place is so bizarre,' said Mick. 'But staying with a family is the best way to do it, because you feel the culture straight away. We stay in too many hotels so it's nice to actually get into the culture, especially here.'

Mama-san bowed, we bowed back, then Mama-san bowed, and we bowed back. Such activities are common in Japan. We didn't know when to stop. Was it rude to stop? We needed to learn such things. This tennis match of bows was won by Mama-san, 5 sets to 3.

We sat — on the ground again — for dinner where a smorgasbord of little chopsticks bordered little plates and bowls containing miso soup, small fried fish, rice, soya beans, seaweed and tempura. Every plate had its own purpose and Mama-san made sure the tide never dropped out of the green tea. Her husband, 'Papa-san', sat in the corner, ready to bow every time we made eye contact. His smile showed he was happy we were there and it made us feel very welcome.

Soon, it was dark and time for bed, but we walked across the road to get an idea of what the waves were like. The ocean doesn't lose its attraction anywhere in the world, and we are never satisfied until we find the place where waves greet the shore. It was very dark, but Mick and I could just make out small waves peaking under the flicker of moonlight. With our bearings in order, we went to the toilet, like any Mama-san would instruct before sleep. It was a hole in the ground. Mick stickered three of his new boards, and then after a series of bows signalling our retirement for the night, our tired travelling bodies became horizontally fused to our futons.

'Oi! You awake?' I guess Mick heard me rolling around, jet-lagged and unable to sleep. When I say that the walls were paper thin, it isn't just an expression; they were actually made of paper. 'Yeah, you too?' No matter how much you travel, jet lag doesn't get any easier. We stretched, waxed boards and talked until the first glimpse of morning, some hours later. We covered everything — relationships, religion, which boards were working, what sort of surfing he wanted to do this week, how we were going to shit in the hole in the ground that was our toilet — all normal topics of conversation when you can't sleep.

Then morning broke. The sun started by warming the back of the mountain, then all of it. It brought indirect light to the village and the surrounding forest before climbing over the mountain and lighting up the surf. The walk to the event site was no more than 500 metres, but in the short time it took us to walk there, word had travelled: Mick Fanning was in town. The scene was hilarious, at least from my point of view.

'Foto, foto, prease … foto.' Before the sun had properly popped, Mick had posed for at least thirty photos, been bowed to several hundred times, and battled through autograph hunters. He couldn't get halfway through a stretch without turning to pose for a photo.

I videoed as Mick was trying out some boards — and in that time a crowd gathered, watching him surf, making mental notes of his make of surfboard and when he decided to swap boards. 'Foto, foto, prease … foto.' There was a group of thirty or so people around me, each new person greeting me with a bow of the head, motioning to the board and the white-headed guy sitting in the line-up. 'Mick Fanning?' They knew exactly who it was but it was more polite to ask than to state.

In between surfs we went to a technical appliance shop. It was as big as an Australian outback town and had things in it that I'd never seen before. But we kept going back for the same reason — the massage chairs. It seems like a simple appliance, but when you sit in a massage chair that is worth around US$20,000, you experience the ultimate in robotic comfort. The managers of the store soon caught on to our little scheme but their heads still bowed, whilst ours were massaged.

Mick won his first heat and we spent the rest of the day discovering the coastline. We found a right bombie and surfed for a couple of hours. Even in the surf, heads bowed and smiles welcomed us where words couldn't. The wave broke pretty far out, and from the ocean, the view was amazing — a rich green landscape, with a rising topography of volcanic mountains dipping into lush valleys. All around us was the old Japan, the real Japan.

That day, a typhoon was developing and the waves were becoming huge. Round three was moved to Malibu, a place where a massive freeway literally goes over the top of the shoreline of the wave. The event structure was set up on the footpath and we prepared for his heat in its shade. The crowd was growing. At one stage, the national sumo champion came to visit. He was helped down the stairs and onto the beach so that he could mingle with the surfing stars. In Japan, sumo wrestling is huge. This guy was a millionaire; married to the finest of Japanese models, and had servants to wipe his arse (as his arm couldn't reach around the fat) and tend to his every need so that he could do what he did best — become fat and move people out of rings with his undies on.

The star at our event was actually of Polynesian blood and good friends with Sunny Garcia, the 2000 World Champion. The ground shook as the sumo champion walked across the sand and his bulk, when compared with Sunny's (who weighs in at around 95 kilograms), was impressive. He had to be the biggest human I'd ever seen. I'm surprised the sheer weight of him didn't implode his bones. And it was through that power and his ability to keep his balanced bulk centred that he remained undefeated. I thought it would be an interesting exercise to count how many bows he received in a day.

When the event started, things became even crazier. I imagine this is what rock stars and David Beckham deal with. The attention Mick, Kelly, Taj and Joel got in Japan was intense, or at least way beyond anything else they had experienced on tour. The crowd continued to grow and the scene was surreal. When Mick won his heat and it was time to leave the beach, we devised a devilish plan to limit his exposure and have a bit of fun. I put his hat on and carried his boards up to the car, pretending to be him. I was his decoy; I enjoyed the game. 'Foto, foto prease,' they beckoned me and I slowly moved to one corner of the highway, lulling them into a false sense of security and identity. During this time, Mick, in my hat and sunnies, with a towel over his head, moved swiftly to the car. I'd be lying if I said it wasn't fun. Using my supreme height advantage, I waited till Mick was safely inside the car before I disappointed his fans with my face. Then one of them said, 'Mick Fanning coach … prease foto, prease.'

For the first time in his life, Mick had to wait while I signed autographs — and I laughed at the irony.

The next day, the final day, Mick lost in the quarters. Leaving the beach became a matter of priority because none of his friends were in the final. This was the year that Andy beat Kelly in the dying seconds, but before that happened, we were on our way to the car and our phones to change our tickets home. Since the mood had changed from happy/cheeky to disappointed, we hadn't prepared our disguises, which up until now had been working well. When Mick crossed the highway to the other side people noticed. One person, then two … Maybe a touch of white hair protruded from under his hat. Three people, twenty-five people … Before you knew it, there was a traffic jam and Mick was in the middle of a moshpit of Japanese signature hunters. Culture shock returned and Mick smiled, surrendering to the Japanese offensive. In the background, the steep mountains were green with life. Below them, a mega highway worked the shoreline, carrying technology to urban life. And in between it all, Mick signed posters amongst bowing heads. All shared the awe.

## DRAGONFLY

Respect is a word that deserves a paragraph. Respect celebrates understanding, breaks up fights, meshes ideas. It is the building block of society. And as Matt Pitts would decide, it is the soul of Japan.

Pittsy, now forty, is an Australian with many connections to Japan. He is a professional surfer-cum-singer/songwriter who just made it into the top 45 — of pop hits in Japan. He's come a long way from his first hit, 'I'm just a train surfer, living in Japan'. He has been living in Japan for over fifteen years and is only now starting to get over the culture shock by learning how to fit in this society of contrasts. He was our chaperone whilst we were in Japan and it was during this time that he told me his story.

'My first trip to Japan was to Najima for an ASP event in 1986,' he recalled, his eyes searching his brain for the dates. 'I went over there by myself and I didn't have a sponsor. It was the year Tom Curren beat Elko in the final. I was kind of trying to make it as a professional surfer, but I was doing it tough. Anyway, I met a local girl. Her name was Yuki Tsunoda and she had a sign saying "I'm homeless, desperate and hungry". I wore the sign as a T-shirt at the contest.' He laughed, 'I didn't even know what it said because it was in Japanese. Anyway, a guy rang me and said, "I have a wetsuit company." The next thing I knew I was flying down to Mizaki and the guy gave me a deal. I got sponsored and ended up staying for a while. I had such a great time. They wanted me to stay longer. I thought I could easily flag the World Tour, do the Japanese domestic tour and make a bunch of money doing it. They kept waving the carrot if I committed to staying full time. So it was a hard decision because it all happened quite quickly.

'I remember being in Hawaii that year, wondering what to do. I was sitting out at Laienikea one day and someone said, "You're doing the tour next year, right?" and I said, "Nah, I'm going to Japan!" I decided right there and then. So I paddled in, rang up United Airlines, took the flight on frequent flyer points and I've been here ever since.

'When I went back to Glen Pang's [Hawaiian shaper] where I was staying, Dog [Richard Marsh, a good friend and former world number 7] asked, "What the fuck are you talking about?" They thought I was on smack! He used to write notes and leave messages around the house saying, "Pittsy, are you all right? You're weird." It was a pretty funny time of my life and it probably was a weird decision, especially because nobody had ever done anything like that before. But it felt right.

'So I went back to Japan and I ended up getting sponsored by this hotel in Mizaki. That was on Tanegashima Island, which is south of Kyushu, on the south island.' What began with a difficult decision became pretty easy: all he had to do was surf. He got free accommodation in the hotel and was looked after quite well. All of a sudden his peers were not questioning his weird decision. 'Man, he was killing it,' recalled Dog. 'We were all grovelling on the tour and here Pittsy was, getting paid good money and he didn't even have to compete.'

'I just had to surf for the hotel.' Pittsy laughed. 'That was it. The boss would ring me and say, "We're having a meeting today, so can you surf from nine to eleven in the morning out the front of the hotel?" And that was it. I was like, "There's a trick, right?" I was getting five to six thousand a month and had to do nothing but surf.'

While most Aussies were battling to get into what was then the top 16, Pittsy was wondering where to put his time and money.

'It set me up financially in Oz which is amazing. Plus I surfed so many great waves. And it was so uncrowded. Japan is the best-kept secret as far as waves and doing what you want goes.'

He might not have been the best on the World Tour, but Pittsy found some silverware pretty quickly on the Japanese domestic circuit.

But it wasn't all smooth sailing. 'I came seventh in the first year on the Japanese ASP Tour and then I won their tour in '95 and '99. I was the first Western guy over there and a lot of the locals were really off me. They devised all these weird rules which made it almost impossible for me to compete. They have some great waves there and a pretty cool vibe — as cool as you can be in a competitive environment anyway. That vibe is why I first struggled to fit in. It was so cutthroat on the World Tour. We had no real sponsors so we had to make prize money; we'd paddle over our own mothers to win. But when you treat the Japanese the same way, they think you're the biggest prick. I would just think, "Well, I'm here to win, not make friends." They thought it was dirty tactics, but it was kind of the way I had grown up in Oz. And when you're on the World Tour, it is the only way to survive.'

Eventually, Pittsy began to mould himself to fit the Japanese way. Around the same time as his transformation, a surprise meeting gave him a further direction.

'I bumped into Damien Oliver [champion Australian jockey] one time in Japan. It was funny because he told me he was a race jockey and I didn't know who he was. So for conversation I asked, "Won any races lately?" He said, "Yeah. The Melbourne Cup." Anyway, he told me how aggressively he was used to riding, doing whatever it took to win a race. He'd been struggling to fit into the Japanese races also and learned just before me that this wasn't the Japanese way. He said, "Now I just get on the horse, whip it and run my race." You just can't do it over here. It's too aggressive for the Japanese lifestyle. It took me a while to find my place.

'There's a line between the Japanese and Australian culture and I felt in between there. I was free and that was awesome. I was learning the language. But the real trip was that I used to live in Japan using my

Aussie head. I'd think that the way they were doing things was wrong, because it was different. Now I've switched my head around and it really makes sense. You think, "Oh my God! They've got it wired." For example, I was with a Japanese friend on the Gold Coast and we noticed that a phone booth had been smashed. My friend asked me what had happened and I explained that some kid must have smashed it. He responded, "Who could be so lacking in common sense to do that?" I thought, "Well, you're right." Some kids beat up someone that same day and he asked what had happened. Again he said, "Why would you do that?"

'There is no crime and violence in Japan and it's one of the things that makes them work as a society. It's a Buddhist lifestyle. They don't intrude on people's space, or interfere, especially in any physical way. We do that in everyday life here in Oz.

'If there's a problem, the boss of the group sorts it out. They'll say, "You're wrong, he's right," and it's over. They have a pecking order on how things work. And boom! It's done. Nobody questions it. You can get groups that have an arsehole as a boss, but generally they are the boss because of their wisdom and experience. The system operates in work and social groups, and in surfing circles there is always the boss in a line-up. The boss role is usually decided by age, as there's a lot of respect for age in Japan. And it works.

'Another awesome thing is the way that the mafia works. They run the country and they are so smart. They'll only sell drugs or arms to people that interest them, not to school kids or young people, so there is no small-time crime or drug problem. I haven't seen drugs the whole time I've been here. None of the kids get exposed to drugs and it's because the mafia keep that world to a level of people who are in control of handling it. It's something that they haven't worked out in Oz yet. In Australia there are too many kids getting on crack, drinking, fighting and stealing. In Japan it's so safe because people are walking around straight. If some small-time dealer came along, the mafia would knock him off because he'd be hurting the kids and the culture.'

Pittsy continued, 'The Japanese culture is still very non-confrontational and it's such a relaxing and comfortable way to live your life. I wish I'd worked that out earlier because now I have a ball. It's a small country but with a massive population. It would be amazing if the rest of the world could work the way they do.

'I've spent the last ten to fifteen years in Japan, learning the language and surfing. I did their tour for about ten years and I'm still up there now, living six months in Japan and six months in Oz. I do the Japanese Web commentary at some of the World Tour events these days and I really feel connected to the place now. I feel like I'm giving back because I get to meet all the kids. You like them; you want to see them do well. Some of them stay at my house in Australia and are getting serious about competition.'

There are some good surfers in Japan but the question remains: why can't they succeed on the World Tour? Pittsy explains.

'You can make great money on the Jap circuit; the average surfer is making ten thousand a month. So they make enough money to not do the World Tour. Aussie kids don't have that choice. The Japanese have a massive population and there is heaps of money in the industry so you can be a rock star in Japan and not have to leave. The money is actually a deterrent. If we could have done that in Oz we wouldn't have left either. That's the hurdle to make them hungry. I don't blame the Japanese. Imagine the Brazilians giving them shit in the heats. This current generation thinks, "Why should we leave the country to get beaten? No thanks." They come up against Brazilians who want to fight him in a heat, threaten to kill them in the car park. Why would they want to deal with that? They've actually got that dream going already, they are already paid money to surf without leaving home.'

But sooner or later someone will have a go at the world title and Pittsy believes the time is near.

'Kato Arashie and Hiroto Arai are both around twelve and probably are the first who have a real chance of making it to the top. Those two kids will make it. They're complete machines at twelve, so ten years from now, the possibilities are looking good. The new generation will have the opportunity and hunger to progress past the current mentality.'

These days, Pittsy is at one with Japan and its culture. The two cultures that before clashed now mesh in mutual respect. Many days when he is sitting in the line-up of Snapper Rocks (where he also lives) he catches himself dreaming of Japan, with memories beckoning him back. Now that he is also fusing his surfing lifestyle with a career in the music industry, he is becoming poetic about his future.

'The landscape is amazing. When you see Mount Fuji at full colour, it's an incredible sight. The cherry blossoms are like coral on land; the hawk hunter is like a firefly. They hover above water and it's like a million soft Christmas lights snaking around riverbeds. There are lots of things I'll never forget. Like how important family is. I spent time with a family. It takes a while to break that barrier, but once you're through, it doesn't matter what's going on, they will never turn you away. If you need to stay with relatives in Oz, they sometimes say, "Sorry, I've got friends staying,

I can't fit you in." Not the Japs.' He laughs. 'They just slot you in beside Grandma.'

The idea of becoming a rock star is also exciting to Pittsy, especially as he climbs the charts. His ability to see Japan through Japanese eyes has helped to give the Japanese a chance to see Australia through his eyes. His connection to Japan started with surfing and now, through his music, they can connect with him.

'It's come full circle and now that I'm doing it again and sitting on the beach playing my guitar, it could be pretty serious. I'm making up songs half in English and half in Japanese. It's happening naturally, I guess because I am sort of half-Japanese and half-Australian now. They're saying the way I put my words together is really interesting, so they're into it. There's one song they really like. It's called "Dragonfly in Heaven". I talk about why my life's charmed; it's more or less the reasons why I live in Japan. I sing about swimming with dolphins, how surfers are sharing that ocean space. It's the Aussie surfer and the new Jap learning how to be non-confrontational together, living in mutual respect.'

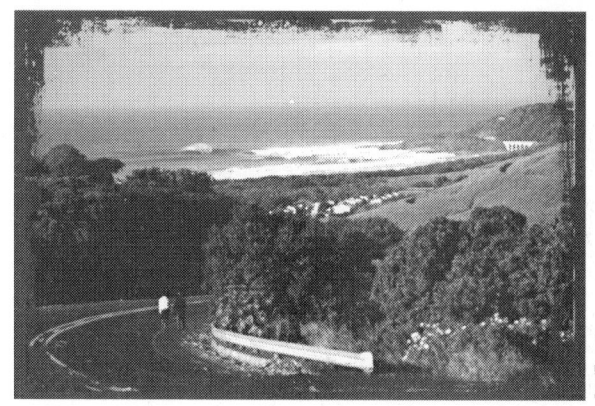

# LIONISE
## SOUTH AFRICA

South Africa is hardcore — beautifully chaotic and raw. On the land are rolling mountains and sunburned plains that are home to animals that can maul you, and snakes and spiders that can poison you. In the water, the Atlantic and Indian oceans wrap around the coast like two bullies separated from a fight. The shores are littered with stories of ill fortune told by the ghosts of the early whalers and explorers come to grief on the optimistically named Cape of Good Hope. Though the dolphins and whales might extend a peaceful invitation, the currents, big waves and, of course, the sharks are testimony to the ocean's danger.

On shore, and in the people's lifestyle and culture, the diversity continues. There is disease that can cripple and kill you and clashing cultures that are fuelled by centuries of struggle. From the tribal cultures, to the British and Dutch colonists, to the North African migrants seeking opportunity, South Africa is still finding its post-apartheid identity. The educated all speak at least three languages, some others speak with clicking sounds — and some don't speak at all.

Beyond the clashes and uncertainty, there is one thing the people have in common. They are all paving the road for a new nation. The following people's stories will tell you about South Africa — where it has been and where it is going. Their stories may offend, inspire, intrigue or challenge you. To understand their stories you need to surrender your judgement to this ancient and beautiful land, with all its social and political volcanoes — Africa's great hope.

## ONE LADY'S FIGHT

Primrose is a lady of exceptional smiles. She comes from the 'shanty town' (what we would call slums) behind Jeffreys Bay and works as a maid in a house on the famous surfing point. Like most coloured people, she makes the one-hour walk twice every day to find work in the rich white township. It was through her job, and his, that Mick Fanning was fortunate enough to meet her. Mick is there every year for the Billabong Pro — Jeffreys Bay is stop six on the World Championship Tour (WCT) and is a favourite for all professionals.

'We just took to her straight away,' said Mick, who first met her in 2003. 'Every day she had the biggest smile on her face. She was so vibrant and I just wanted to hug her, be around her and talk to her. I'd come in from surfing every day and ask if she wanted a cup of tea. We'd just sit and talk for a while. I loved it.'

Primrose has a story that isn't too uncommon in this country. She has AIDS, in a place where one in three people suffer from the disease. If you exclude the five million whites who live in the country (relatively few of whom have contracted AIDS), you could say that of the rest of the population — the forty million blacks — almost half have it.

'Primrose told us that social workers used to come to the shanty towns and teach them the practice of safe sex,' said Mick. 'They would use a carrot to demonstrate how to roll on a condom and told the people that if they used these condoms, no-one would get sick anymore. The next day, the social workers came in to check on their progress, and one of the men proudly showed them a carrot wrapped in a condom that he had put on his bedside table before he had sex. He thought he was safe.'

At first, the blacks believed that the white people were telling them not to have sex, or insisting they practise safe sex as a way of population control, so they mistrusted their teachings. Now, AIDS itself is ultimately a form of population control. Basically, the problem stems from a lack of education. For example, when the former South African spokesperson for AIDS was in court on a rape charge, he was later acquitted because the judge believed that the woman consented. When asked if he was concerned about AIDS, he replied that he wasn't worried about contracting the deadly disease from this lady, who he knew had the virus, because he took a shower after sex.

We, especially Mick, got to know Primrose quite well during the time we spent at J-Bay. Halfway through a cup of tea one day, she told us her story: three men raped her one night, which is how she contracted the disease. Unfortunately, her story is way too common in South Africa. She later became pregnant, and when she lost her child at five months of age, found out that the child died because she had AIDS and had passed it on to her baby. What a way to find out you have AIDS: by losing a son. Your first! His photo sleeps on the bed with her every night.

'It is so tough,' said Mick who, along with his mum Liz, sends Primrose money for medicine — and invests just as much time and emotional support in the form of phone calls and emails.

One day Primrose invited us to her home to go to church and listen to the men sing, an event which was the pride of the town. We were honoured to be invited to this special cultural experience. It was a Sunday and driving in to the town was like breaching the walls of an alien world. The clean wheels of our white hire car hit the black dust — and the differences began. Houses were made of corrugated iron and leaned on each other in a twisted mess of metal, wire and wood. Some had roofs, some didn't; some had electricity, but most didn't. In their dirt yards, fires burned the rubbish from the previous day, sending forth thick black smoke. There were no schools and no tradesmen but still, a society exists with its own shops and workers. The post-apartheid vision of blacks and whites living side by side appears to be just an idea as you wouldn't bump into a white person in this shanty town. Throughout the town, mums hung out the washing on fishing line, while their kids played war games with sticks, and football with something they had found in the bin.

Then we arrived at the Christian church, which was the best building in the town thanks to generous donations and strong belief. We waited outside the church until several men in robes and their children walked across the road and gathered in a circle to sing and dance. The magic of the rhythm and harmony they produced far exceeded that of musical instruments and they sang with a rich passion and pride. In their culture, there is much uncertainty, but they have always had their singing — and they share it beautifully. Looking around, you realised that Primrose, who had stolen our hearts, was only one of many who shared the same story. Gunk wrestled the corners of the kids' eyes; spots and blemishes marked their beautiful skin — a reminder of the disease that was killing them from the inside out.

'There are so many people here that need help,' said Mick, who leaves a whole quiver of boards and clothes with the kids of this town every year. 'But Primrose has had a personal effect on me, you know? You can't help everyone, but you can help the people that have had an impact on your life in some way. She's always smiling and laughing and just has the biggest heart. She's my friend and amazing and I'd do whatever I can for her.'

In 2006, Primrose still worked in the house. Her body showed signs of weakness and her eyes had developed a blinding layer of film, suggesting an outcome we weren't ready to face. At times, she would stop work and sit on the balcony with us to cheer Mick on. Mick ended up winning an event over Taj Burrow and, with a portion of his first place prize money, paid for her to have a sight-saving eye operation. She can see properly again now and has stopped having headaches, but unfortunately, there is no happy ending with AIDS.

In 2007, Primrose used Mick's money to set up a centre where people could learn computer techniques, but the place was robbed and all the computers were stolen. She then opened a hairdressing salon next to her house in the shanty town. We went in there for a haircut when a young woman was having hair extensions put in. 'She is blind,' explained Primrose. 'She can't see her hair so she wants to feel it.' We had our own hair extended for laughs. Outside, kids played happily in the twilight. Life was good — or so it seemed.

The next day, Primrose sat in our house crying, something she rarely did. Her cousin had just lost her five-month-old child in a car crash — and the tears flooded down her face. 'My baby was five months too!' We hugged each other and wondered when it would all end.

When the surf trip had drawn to a close, Primrose gave Mick a photo of her son to give to his mum, who still carries it in her wallet. But Primrose is not one who concentrates on the adversity in life. When we sat down for tea on the last morning with her, neither the disease nor the emotional goodbye from a special friend could hide the smile coming from the amazing soul within her. We all hugged. Nobody wanted to let go.

## THREE PROS

Greg Emslie is from East London. It's an older coastal town which has, like Greg himself, a youthful energy and a global attraction. It's a town a lot of people go to on their way to Cape Town or J-Bay, but not a town that a lot of people leave. Greg, however, has had reason to leave, thanks to his skill on a surfboard. At thirty, you would have to call him the senior member of the South African elite. He has won a World Junior Title (1994) and has been competing in the top 45 for longer than any other countryman since their first world champion, Shaun Thomson (1977). I sat with Greg and his peers for a chat on a lay day during the Nova Schin Pro in Brazil to talk about everything South African.

'We are a very competitive nation,' said Greg. 'The South African surfers are starting to believe in themselves and in their surfing ability. The numbers are getting bigger and we are definitely capable of producing more world champions.'

Greg's friends often stop by in East London on their pilgrimage to J-Bay, staying at his father's bed and breakfast in town. The raw countryside of South Africa is an amazing sight to behold. 'It's a great little city,' said Greg. 'It takes five minutes to get anywhere, the people are relaxed and very friendly, the pubs serve ice-cold beer and there are always some fun waves to be had. Being a smaller city we have a tight-knit community. I feel a lot safer there than in the big cities. The townsfolk also cherish life and enjoy the fun parts of life.'

Greg's observation about safety is an interesting point. As you travel west, there are generally more whites — with more money and more security. But, although there are still some social and political problems in these small towns, Greg remains positive about their future.

'Lots of people have left South Africa and were negative about the place. Now a lot of them are coming back. The new South Africa has been very up and down in the last ten years, as you would expect. But things have settled down in the last two to three years and now it is a place of opportunity. Everyone has had to learn to adapt and make things happen. It has all been a great part of growing our rainbow nation.'

But not everyone shares Greg's positivity about social issues. Former Durban pro, Byron Howarth, has already moved to Australia, feeling unsafe in his own country. 'I love the country and I love the waves. South Africa is such a special place, but when I left I'd had enough. My girlfriend had been mugged — it just isn't a safe place anymore.' Byron moved to Byron Bay where he now works for Electric Sunglasses, and his girlfriend has never felt safer. 'To live in a house where you don't have to have barbed wire fences and being able to walk around at any time — you guys don't know how lucky you are. I love Australia and this is how I want to live,' she declared.

Travis Logie is one of the new breed leading the latest charge, including names like Davie Weare, Ricky Basnett, Royden Bryson and their new world amateur champion, Jordy Smith. Travis, a world amateur champion in 2001, is also from Durban — a place that epitomises post-apartheid South Africa. It houses the largest Indian population outside of India, a flash flood of Northern African immigrants, a stubborn Afrikaans minority. Picture an old rich holiday town like Surfers Paradise; now strip away the infrastructure that keeps the town clean and functioning and in five years you'd have Durban — arguably the most dangerous city in the world. But if you look deeper, there are some amazing pockets and, like any city, it offers excitement, opportunity, and consistent waves for up-and-coming surfers.

'It's a super fun city,' said Travis. 'And the waves are fun and consistent. When you grow up there, you know where to go and where not to go, so I feel relatively safe.'

Durban is where most of the surfers and the related industry come to. Five piers hold the sand in place, so the ocean doesn't wash away the holiday and apartment buildings that tower up to twenty storeys high on the shoreline. Here the sun rises at six, but it isn't until lunchtime that it makes the climb over the buildings, leaving many a dark corner for shady operations.

Indians, English, Dutch, and many Northern Africans from places like Zimbabwe, Nigeria and the Congo have made the journey south since Nelson Mandela became president of the new Republic of South Africa. They came looking for work opportunities, but often found them through crime. Every day, 4000 illegal immigrants cross the borders into South Africa, some of whom end up in the belly of lions as they walk through Kruger National Park to

Johannesburg. By consuming so much human flesh, the lions have even contracted human-borne viruses such as pneumonia.

The stories about South Africa flood as fast as the immigrants.

'Since the blacks took power, they have turned everything around,' said Travis. 'People from Northern African nations — the Nigerians, the Congolese and the Zimbabweans — are looking for opportunity but quickly turn to crime. They run the drug trade and rule street crime. They have no regard for life. They would kill someone for a pair of sneakers, I'm telling you, bru. The dangerous thing is that before they commit a crime, they often perform a month of rituals involving their culture's witch doctors. They drink potions, dance around and attempt a robbery thinking they are bullet proof.

'Just recently in Durban, some blacks robbed a cash carrier. They took the money and made their getaway, but they threw kerosene on the drivers of the car and burned them alive. Now the cash carriers have police guards but they are in on it too, for a cut of the money. So it's all just fucked up!

'When you talk about the future the hard thing for us is the uncertainty. My girl has forty million rand worth of farm property up north. Soon it will be subdivided and houses will be built making it worth over 100 million. But who's to stop the blacks from coming in and "land grabbing", like they did in Zimbabwe?' Since Mandela became president, there have been many examples of native blacks seizing land, and killing and driving the white farmers off land they had owned for generations.

Travis has even seen a lot of changes on his own beachfront. 'For example, you would never see a white beggar five years ago. Now they are everywhere on the beachfront at Durban. I'm telling you, I feel so lucky that I have a British passport. If it gets unsafe for me and my family, I'm out of there.'

We were sitting at a bar having this conversation and straight away Greg took offence. 'Well, why don't you just go now!' said Greg. 'You have to stand by your country and fight for what you believe in.' The tribal elder had spoken. But the debate will continue.

## THE BEST RIGHT IN THE WORLD

In complete contrast to Durban, J-Bay is the most beautiful place in the world. You can't help but give in to the mellow vibe that overwhelms the long bay. Whales float by, dolphins catch waves and barrels and perfect swells rhythmically chase the point three kilometres down into a bay that looks like a moving oil painting.

The days of endless summer, when travelling hippies ran over the sand dunes to surf empty waves, are now gone but the feeling has stayed — and not even the thousands of houses on the hill can change that. For years there was even a hippy who lived in the undergrowth of the brush on the point. He cut himself a little cave in the thick brush and lived a simple life as a resident squatter. He was there for so long that he actually had legal rights to stay there.

'That guy was radical,' said Mickey Lindsay, who works for Billabong in the surf industry town. 'The full Herman. He'd come out and surf, then go back in his little shell. I guess too many surfers spoilt the serenity of his decade-long sanctuary — and nobody has seen him since.'

Mickey made the move from Durban and settled down with his family in Cape St Francis. 'It's such a peaceful little town and a great place for the kids to grow up. The point pumps and there are beachies everywhere.'

Like most of South Africa, the coastline here is raw and beautiful. 'Life is so much better for us here,' said Micky. 'We've just gone from a rat race with crime and safety issues, to a place where the kids can play on the street and we can leave the door unlocked. It's magic. Plus the waves are so much better. When J-Bay is on, there is nothing like it.'

'It's got to be one of the best waves in the world,' said Jake Paterson, who twice won the Billabong Pro there. 'But the good waves come with cold weather. When the polar bears [surf speak for cold weather] are coming, you know the waves are too, so it's a bit more hardcore than anywhere else. But the rewards are there.'

There are a series of five points, starting at Boneyards and going all the way down to Albatross. When it works, your chin will drop and dribble — there are not many places equal to J-Bay.

## BLACK MAN DON'T SURF

While in France in 2006, a journalist approached me requesting an interview with Mick Fanning. This was nothing unusual, but after speaking with him for an hour or two, I realised he was an interesting guy. He had grown up in New York City, and then lived in Paris. He had just come back from Lebanon where he had been covering the war for the major Parisian press. Several people a day want to interview Mick, and my job consists more of managing them than building his profile. However, I mentioned to Mick that an interview with this journalist might be interesting, because I thought he was going to ask some unusual questions instead of talking about the exact same stuff that every journalist does. This reporter didn't surf and wouldn't know how to put a wettie on the right way. If you gave him a board, he'd probably wax the bottom and paddle out backwards. But his first question to Mick knocked him for six.

'I want to know why black people don't surf.'

Just think about that question for one minute … And it applies to every country, not just Africa. A few possible answers — but in the form of more questions — spring to mind: are blacks not accepted into the white-dominated line-up? Is our purist sport that relishes in the freedom associated with nature's ocean too expensive for the economically challenged? Are they just not ocean people?

There are no real answers here, only opinions and more questions.

'Coloured people have generally been brought up playing physical sports such as soccer, rugby, athletics and boxing,' said Greg Emslie. 'I think over time they will become more interested in water sports and with this the surfing culture will develop.'

Some black kids are starting to surf at J-Bay and Durban, thanks to donations from pros like Mick Fanning, but it's only happened in recent years.

Lack of social acceptance can also be a big deterrent. Just ask any girl who attempted surfing in the eighties and early nineties. Now women are everywhere! Will the same explosion happen once the floodgates of acceptance open for black surfers? Racial acceptance should not still be an issue, but unfortunately in South Africa it is.

And that reporter's question could also be asked about the dark corners of many other activities.

## SHARK HUNTER

I once interviewed an amazing person during my time at *Tracks* surfing magazine — a shark researcher from Natal who had recently been photographed swimming with Great Whites in a shot that made the cover of the magazine. However, he wasn't just swimming with them; he was actually riding them, hanging on to their dorsal fin, looking back at the camera and mocking everything we fear. I was unsure of the ratio of lunacy and wisdom flowing through his veins, but upon talking to him, I discovered that it was his wisdom that led to his bold attempt to prove that sharks don't eat humans. While he didn't get eaten, the imagery suggested that the shark was the one who made the decision. The photographs are spooky. Picture it — a six-foot-tall man, with his arms reaching two to three feet in front of him to grab the dorsal fin (itself three feet high), and his flippers, also two to three foot long, didn't even reach the shark's tail. It had to be six metres. I'll never forget his response to one question I asked him, 'What do you do if you see a shark coming?'

'Don't run,' he said. 'A shark's prey will always run. That's how it identifies food.'

You need to be a certain type to take on nature here in South Africa. One such man is Andrew Carter, who has been surfing here for over two decades. He is a hardcore surfer who travels from coast to coast looking for the best possible waves with no-one else out on them. You'll often find him chasing swells through the Transkei, an independent nation of rolling hills, perfect waves and the odd shanty town with no medical facilities. Like any South African surfer, he is aware of the chances he takes and on 9 July 1994 at around lunchtime, he found himself sharing the line-up with his worst fears.

'I was surfing at Nahoon Reef in East London when, without any warning, I felt a huge impact on my left,' he recalled. 'I turned and came face to face with a large Great White. It had me and my board clamped in its jaw, and it felt like it was crushing my legs. I recall its tremendous power; it felt like I was in a giant vice. Luckily it opened its mouth to get a better bite and I rolled out of the way. The next bite missed me and munched into my board. I managed to swim some metres away while it went moggy, chewing my board. I realised I was a long way from the beach and bleeding badly, so I knew I had little chance without some flotation. I turned to see the shark release my board and slip back into the waves. I decided my best bet was to get back to the board and thus have something to fend off another attack. Then the luckiest wave of my life arrived and I managed to turn the bitten board around and bellyride the wave back to safety.

'Unfortunately, the shark turned on another surfer nearby, severing his leg just below the knee. He died in hospital later that day. I escaped with around 500 stitches and staples internally and externally. I have a large jaw-shaped scar that runs from my knee to my hip. Luckily I only lost a little amount of flesh, as that is what causes problems later. I know I have about 80 per cent use of my leg and can still manage a half-decent off the top, but most importantly, pulling into the barrel is still okay.'

You'd think an episode like this would deter — or at least curb — his adventurous spirit, but Andrew knows no other way to live. 'I certainly have my shark radar going full tilt when I'm out surfing, but I still surf the same spot and sometimes find myself sitting on my own in the same place that I was attacked. Mad maybe — but the reef is the spot for good surf 70 per cent of the time. As for talking about sharks, that's no problem. It's probably therapeutic. The ocean is the sharks' domain so I guess it's their place to feed. I would just prefer it if it wasn't me they fed on.'

## THE GARDEN ROUTE

It's regarded as one of the best drives in the world: the N2 from Port Elizabeth to Cape Town, where the world's natural wonders rise and fall from the wild, undulating landscape. Along the way are green hills sprinkled with yellow flowers and rising mountains and cutting gorges where rivers slither to the sea. We got to experience one such gorge with a piece of bungy cord tied to our ankles, freefalling 216 metres into a canyon. I've done sky diving before, and I've bungy-jumped from a hundred feet, but nothing can prepare you for this. It's the world's biggest. Even the second freefall after you bounce is bigger than anything else in the world. If you're in town — do it!

For six hours, the road between J-Bay and Cape Town dazzles and surprises you. The earth takes you in and you start to understand the African connection to the land. During the journey I stopped in at a quiet little country town called Wilderness, just near George. My host was Sean Holmes, probably South Africa's most talented surfer, who has won everything from national titles and WQS events to the Red Bull Big Wave Challenge at Dungeons in Cape Town. He was also Andy Irons' nemesis at J-Bay for a few years where he received a wildcard, beating the then world champ two years in a row. At thirty, Sean exudes a humility and peacefulness that is rooted in the fertile sands of his homeland. When I met him on this trip, he had just quit his job at Billabong to remove himself from the 'scene' of the surf industry at J-Bay, which really didn't suit him.

'The waves around here are so incredible! Coming from J-Bay, where it gets pretty crowded ... here, I need to find people to surf with. Because of the big mountains we have our own weather system and there is always somewhere going off.'

We surfed Vic Bay — just Sean, myself and his fiancée, Shona. She was an incredible lady. A competitor in skydiving, she is a full-on adrenalin junkie. The waves were six foot and she was charging the sets next to the rock. 'She worries me sometimes,' admitted Sean, who enjoys surfing the biggest waves and swims with sharks when he's spearfishing giant tuna around the reef and points. I was actually glad to get out of there before I got roped into base-jumping the mountain, or spear fishing a Great White!

Back on the road, and about four hours later, the mountains grew more rugged as we approached the Atlantic side of the wild coast and Cape Town. Where the southern peninsula's national park points like a finger to the Antarctic, the mountains drop suddenly — and the two great oceans meet. The park boasts zebras, wild buck, baboons and more, and is only minutes from the city. No matter how big this city grows, it will forever answer to the natural environment — the mountains and the wild coast. When you're at the Cape of Good Hope, you feel like you're at the edge of the world. The finger of land drops deep into the ocean. On your right is the Atlantic, wild and cold; on your left is the Indian Ocean, also wild and cold.

We were just about to surf inside False Bay when a massive swell cornered the Cape, funnelling six to eight foot waves into a protected corner. About ten kilometres straight out was a massive seal colony where sharks dive out of the water to feed and put on shows for documentary and *National Geographic* cameras. It's a hard place to surf, full of giant kelp, sharks and weather. It takes a certain type of maniac with an appreciation for the rawer things in life. That man is Ross Lindsay, my friend and guide.

Ross moved to Cape Town from East London in '84. He owns a casting agency in town, sells blanks, other surf hardware and a shark shield — a new device that sends off electrical impulses to warn off sharks. 'It works like a fire does for humans: when you get close enough, you have to turn away.' In Cape Town, business for shark shields is brisk. 'It doesn't suit surfers as much because it is still a little too heavy; it's more for divers,' he explained. Ross and I surfed away around the peninsula, keeping our eye on Dungeons, a wave now famous for big wave surfers. Ross had been surfing and towing it for a decade or so.

'There's a pretty solid group of hardcore surfers around here,' he told me. 'To get waves, you have to put up with cold water, lots of wild wind and seas, giant kelp — and you have to drive a long way to find them.' We're not talking about seaweed, we're talking about tree-like branches of kelp that move up and down with the rise and fall of swells, creeping up your legs, breaking fins and leaving you high and dry when the water sucks out. It was all a bit too much for me, leaving me feeling spoiled as a surfer and wondering if I'd put up with it myself.

## POLITICS

Talking about South African politics is like opening a can of worms. But these issues have to be faced by us all, surfers or otherwise. However, rather than giving my opinion, I am going to quote the people who live and breathe in this system. It's easy for us to judge, but we should probably spend more time trying to understand before voicing our thoughts.

'Desmond Tutu, the archbishop of basically the whole country, is starting to come out now and say that the people are going too far,' said Davie Weare, a pro surfer from Durban. 'He is saying that the white people gave us [black South Africans] power — and that we shouldn't reverse a situation that was created by whites three generations ago. The politicians are trying to lead the way in giving power back to the people but they are showing the wrong example and taking it too far.'

We were sitting on the beach, back in Brazil. Things were starting to get a little heated. Then we got on to our next topic ... the quota system.

It was a conversation that started with cricket. It's one of South Africa's biggest sports and the people turn to it for hope when their society has none. Regrettably, South Africans are no longer winning the sport in which they used to be world champions. The quota system brought in since Mandela means that a certain percentage of blacks have to be employed in every workplace, including professional sports, in order to create equal opportunity.

'But they aren't educated yet, and don't have the skills to do most jobs. In cricket, the government now believes that there have to be seven blacks in the run-on side [there are eleven in a cricket side]. Mandela's theory is that there are forty million blacks and only five million whites, so the ratio should be the same in the workplace and in professional sport. I'm telling you, bru, the best black athletes get so much money. They get busted for drugs and other things, but they never get sacked because they are so rare and valuable,' said Travis.

'I can't believe we can't get a good Indian spin bowler,' he added, getting back to the argument with an attempt at humour. 'They are half the population in Durban and the biggest Indian population outside India, but we can't find one. Fuck!'

The white South Africans are used to winning and used to getting their own way. The quota system is just one example of a situation where they will have to come to grips with a new government and the reality that they are, in fact, the minority. The new generation of South Africans will live through a very interesting time.

Like their distant predecessors who started their journey in a place called Gondwanaland, it will take a certain tenacity, compassion and rugged appreciation of nature to continue the journey and play their part in what Greg Emslie calls their 'Flowering Nation'.

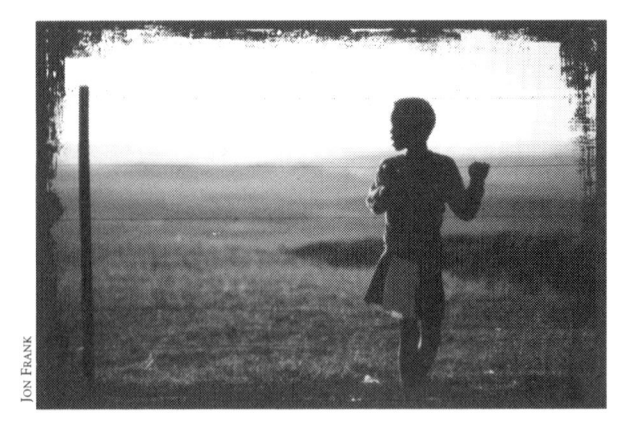

# THE BUSINESS WAS SURVIVAL
## THE TRANSKEI

We were warned not to do it. 'It's too dangerous. Life is cheap there. There are no police. If your car breaks down you're fucked. Make sure you fill up with petrol before you go, and leave early, so you get there before the sun goes down; leave your windows up; don't stop for anyone and don't stop until you get to the other side …'

I must admit the warnings scared us a little, especially since they came from everyone who caught wind of our planned adventure through what they call the 'Wild Coast'. But we went anyway: in defiance of ideas that we thought were based on fear and racism. The car was packed, boards were on the roof and we headed southwest from Durban on the N2, straight into the Transkei, South Africa.

The Transkei, which means 'the area beyond the Kei River', is a region situated on the eastern cape of South Africa. It is also the name of an apartheid-era Bantustan. A Bantustan is an area set aside for blacks for the purpose of concentrating their numbers in one spot.

Nelson Mandela was born there, but he has long since gone. The country has since grown wild — hence its name, hence the warnings.

Naivety is the bedfellow of all young travellers. It is defined as 'having or showing an excessively simple and trusting view of the world and human nature, often as a result of youth and inexperience'.

Youth and inexperience were both on our side when we made the decision to drive through the Transkei. Kieren Perrow, Andy King and myself were trying to get to J-Bay on the other side and couldn't afford air tickets, so we drove through the area that extends from Durban to East London — a distance of around 600 kilometres. It is a place that draws similar warnings from all South Africans. It starts with a deep breath, then is followed with '... beautiful country, but ...' and then come the warnings.

We were excited and scared, but mostly naive. We were only nineteen and it was our first year on tour. Travel was not a word we were learning; it was an experience we were living. And with it, as a natural evolution, came the gathering of intelligence that is multiplied by activities that expose you to people and places unlike your own.

As naive travellers, you don't think that somebody could kidnap you, hijack your car or cut your throat because there might be some nice white money in your pocket. That wouldn't happen where you're from, so why would it happen here?

I find the word 'travel' is a bit of an understatement. 'Travel.' It doesn't even sound very exciting. It should have at least two more syllables and a cool sound that adds mystery and excitement. I bet in the Transkei there's a clicking sound attached to it.

## THE TRANSKEI

Most South Africans will avoid the Transkei altogether. If they do go, there are rules. We heard them all and, for the most part, adhered to them. You have to remember that in 1997, when we travelled there, it was only three years since the end of apartheid, and there was still mistrust, contempt, hatred and a lot of other negative attitudes. We had seen it in Durban but thought that since we didn't feel racist towards them, why would they have a problem with us? Naive!

The first part of the drive was incredibly scenic, and we couldn't just experience it through closed windows. Though we left the motor running, we got out of the car several times to wonder at the Wild Coast, taking pictures, in awe of the power of nature. The rolling hills and gorges, the rivers running out into the coastline where sharks gather in numbers … it was stunning. I heard there are epic waves there. You could even see clean swells approaching the endless bays and beaches, but surfing wasn't on our mind.

Again, what intrigues me is that one minute you're driving past expensive hotels and affluent cafes and houses in Durban and then you cross a border. The landscape is still the same, but you quickly learn that it is not the landscape that makes it 'wild', but the nature of the people. About twenty minutes into the journey we saw people walking on the road and we wondered where they were going.

Many kilometres later, we saw a little shanty town on a hill. It was mostly clay dwellings, with smoke from their fires and the occasional goat searching the parched earth for something green. The people were going about their business. Their business was survival — and they did it in a wild way. There were little stores every now and then, but I'm not even sure if the people had money to buy anything. Unable to interact, we couldn't find out more.

These shanty towns made South Africa's ones look like luxury hotels. Some had thatched roofs, some had corrugated iron that wind and time had twisted and torn from their foundation of rusty nails and rope. They build homes like birds build nests, gathering whatever materials are available to them, found in nature or left on the road — and squeeze all their eggs into the one basket.

Of course, there are no condoms and no education about reproduction, so the women move with babies attached to their every spare part.

The people we saw walking were probably visiting witch doctors in other towns, or just simply roaming. There is no such thing as education, government, policing of the streets or town planning. It was simply wild people living in a wild land, forgotten, untouched. South Africa was the only international country that recognised the Transkei's independence. But since the Transkei didn't want independence, it has become a sort of black hole in the African mindset.

Travellers are warned to take heed in the Transkei region. Any website or travel book would agree. The high incidence of violent crime has turned this into a notorious area, generally avoided by many South Africans. Shootings and armed robberies are frequent in its capital, Umtata. Unfortunately, the N2, the only thoroughfare through the region, leads straight into the heart of it. We experienced this a few hours into our journey.

In some way, we believed on a personal level that we had dealt with racism. In the Transkei, it is rife. There are no white people living there. White people are just the people who drive the colourful expensive cars through their homeland, never helping, never stopping. Suspicion leads to mistrust, which leads to violence.

Up until this point it had been mostly a pleasant drive. The wild nature of the place, combined with the time it had taken, had led to interesting car conversations. We were trying to make sense of these alien ideas. We honestly wondered why people would do something to you unprovoked, just because of the colour of your skin. How naive we were. We believed in the human race and, coming from a place where we held no contempt for black people, thought that they would see that we were good people and to be trusted. We thought we could talk our English, walk into shops with our expensive clothes and connect to people who, across the border in South Africa, still had to walk on the other side of the road from white people.

We stopped a couple of times to take photos and appreciate in silence the beautiful landscape. In all directions, it was only coast, filled with hills and rivers. Every now and then, little communities of clay dwellings added a human element to the wild coast. We had no human interaction of note. Then we entered Umtata.

Usually people walking on the roads indicated that a village was nearby. As we started seeing hundreds of people walking, we figured we were getting close. 'Don't stop the car, even for a red light,' we were warned. I honestly didn't get it. Anyway, we came to our first red light. 'What do we do?' asked Kieren, who at the time was behind the wheel.

'We'll be sweet,' said Andy.

I smiled at some passers-by on the street, a gesture of awareness and acceptance. But what was I accepting? What was I aware of? Within five seconds of stopping at this light a bottle came crashing into our car, smashing into a thousand pieces on the pavement. If the trajectory were a little higher, it would have smashed our windscreen. We didn't know where it had come from, but we couldn't hide from where it was directed. Kieren hit the gas and sped through the red light — and many more until we got out the other side.

We completed the rest of the trip without stopping, but without pushing the car too much for fear of breaking down on the side of the road. We drove past beautiful rivers and mountains, past fields of wild grass with all the colours the soil can give. We drove past a coastline that looked as if it had amazing waves. And we didn't stop once. We weren't naive anymore. However, we hoped that one day we could come to a place like this, communicate with the people, share some stories, some waves and not get eaten by sharks, racism or fear. It introduced us to some realities — to things you can read in a name; things you can get warned about; things you thought you had dealt with as humans. Somewhere in between all this is the 'Wild Coast'.

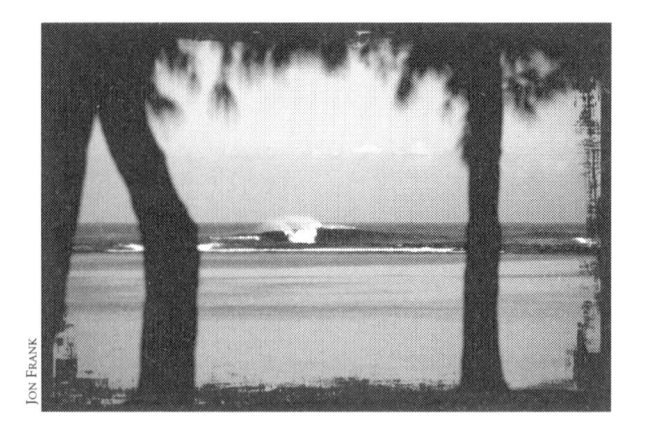

# PLACE D'AFRIQUE
## REUNION ISLAND

Most places seem to adhere to balance. I offer Indonesia as an example. On the yin side you've got perfect waves, beautiful water and weather. On the yang side you've got tsunamis, earthquakes and sea-lice. If you go to the Amazon jungle you'll be swatting flies and bugs and spiders while contemplating the beauty beyond their grip. If you go to the super bank on the Gold Coast, its crowds build a fence in front of the perfection. If you go to Bells or J-Bay, it is the cold that brings balance to these red hot waves. If you go to Reunion Island, there are sharks — mostly tigers. Now we know as surfers that we are unlikely to get eaten, but here you can actually see them. That's the yang. However, Reunion Island seems a place that Mother Nature has spent a while nurturing and there's plenty of yin to balance it.

## SEARCHING

'Hmm, looks good. I like it.' Rip Curl founder Doug 'Claw' Warbrick had just arrived at the point and was regarding the new trophy as if it were his child. It was a colourful, beautifully crafted globe of the world, that spun, as globes do, with tripping suggestion. 'Looks sick,' said Mick Fanning, feeling it in his hands for the first time. Behind us workers were busying themselves like ants, putting together the final touches of the first ever Rip Curl Search WCT, Reunion Island, 2005, while in front of us, a perfect five-foot swell grabbed everyone's attention. It wrapped around the point, growing down the line into a six-foot, rippable wall that drew everyone's thoughts. Like that swell, the idea of the Search WCT had been gathering momentum for a while and had finally come to rest on the shore here at St Leu.

Around the time the world of competitive surfing became a two-tiered system in '91, you may remember a few ASP events at Reunion. If not, you may remember the country from a section in Billabong's *Pump*, where Occy did some of the best surfing, still to this date, ever seen in a video. If you're still not sure where it is, you'll find the island in the southern hemisphere, about 200 kilometres southeast of Mauritius. It's a French province, a place where volcanoes have jumped out of the blue water, where historic cultures sip Bordeaux wine and the wine makers wear ancient jewellery of African origin while speaking French. Being an island, it is also home to some amazing waves — St Leu especially. That is a wave that can make you crazy. It has it all; but, as one local found out, it will eventually bring you balance.

## TARZAN

Tarzan is the gnarly local. He's the guy who always paddles past you, always drops in, talks really loud, builds fires in his eyes and burns you with his look. Everyone has a nemesis when they surf. At Reunion, he is everyone's nemesis. I had encountered him twice, first in '97, then again in 2005 when we came back for the Rip Curl Search WCT. He didn't talk, he just growled. He rode waves at St Leu with animalistic flair and aggression, hence the nickname. What was worse, he rode a Mal. At Reunion, the line-up is ruled by Malibus, bodyboarders and sharks, so it's hard to get used to a foreign pecking order, where one's comfort zones are tested.

Recently, I heard a story about Tarzan. It was told by a French friend who had just been to Reunion on his way back to Australia. We were drinking coffee in my home town of Cronulla and talking about the world, as you tend to do with travellers. 'There is this guy Tarzan from Reunion Island,' he said. I knew exactly who he was talking about, and we compared some stories before he concluded.

'He has been surfing for thirty years like this. He catches any wave he wants. He is really aggressive in the water and on the waves. And he will only surf St Leu. Just last year he started a surf school to teach people how to surf. Now he has to talk to people. He has to go to the hotel where the tourists stay, shake their hands, say welcome, and take them surfing at St Leu and be friendly. He has to be friendly to all the people in the water now too.' As he was telling the story, my best mate and I laughed. 'Everyone can be bought,' we said.

'Yeah, and now that he has become commercial, he has realised that in all those years, he made no friends in the water. He didn't know anywhere outside of St Leu and he had led a closed life. Now he is friends with people from all around the world; he can travel. Now he is a really happy, smiling person. It's cool.'

## THE GURU AND THE FIRE

Tom Curren, who spearheaded the Search in the early nineties, was back at Reunion in 2005 to help lead the Search WCT. This time, though, the three-time world champ was a wildcard. His lines were pure, his style unrelenting. Being back on the program and competing again has also lent more speed to Tom's surfing. His board choice in this event was a six foot six inches remake of his 'black beauty'. It was an emotional and inspiring board, but too long to have much power in the four-foot waves for today's criteria. He spent the rest of the week playing music and chasing waves in the way he remembered the Search. But a long tail of photographers wagged behind him everywhere he went. Even at forty, for Tom, some things never change. As long as he stands on his board with more style and flow than any other, he can ride whatever he wants, play whatever he wants and say whatever he wants. With three world titles under his belt and because he is still a better free surfer than most, it's no wonder he barely speaks. He has nothing left to say.

But when he does talk, you listen. And this week, he was talking a lot about Mick Fanning. Over the years, Tom has had some interesting and always effective advice for Mick in his pursuit of a world title. As Mick's pit boss, I get a lot of people offering me their opinions; it's part and parcel of my job. But what Tom has said from time to time, I will always cherish. This week, he didn't need to say much.

'I don't know which one to ride; they're all sick,' said Mick the night before the event started. He had that same look he had on the Goldy —

nothing fazed him, nobody bothered him, and he was in his own little zone and more focused than ever. The board problem (what a problem to have) was the only hurdle Mick had along the way in this event. When he is in this state of mind he doesn't talk much, but exudes this intense focus. He keeps to himself, talks with himself and surfs for himself. Nobody tried harder, yet surfed as effortlessly as Mick — and he meticulously devoured people all the way to the final.

The waves for the whole event were pumping — clean four to six foot with the occasional bigger set. This wave is so rippable and with almost every surfer doing massive turns, flowing together for the whole ride without stopping or starting — or, heaven forbid, getting caught for a fraction of a second — was crucial. This was something Mick had been working on. When he floated through the fast section, hitting the end bowl and launched into a reo, followed by a massive grab-rail bottom turn and one of the biggest hacks you could ever see, his job was done. He went past my view as caddy and all I could see was fins and spray. When the cheers subsided, the 9.7 was heard. Mick, perhaps the fittest on tour, was racing out the back, legs kicking, arms reaching. He didn't look or think about that trophy once until it sat next to him. When he finally lifted it above his head, he had the world in his hands in more ways than one.

## DON'T GO CHASING WATERFALLS

The next day, we cruised around the island. We hadn't seen very much because we had been focusing on the event, so now it was our time to discover the island. Nathan Hedge and Jonny Frank had a ride in a helicopter.

'It was incredible,' said Hog. 'We were checking all these surf spots that roads can't get to because of the big volcanic mountains. It was pumping! Jonny took some shots and then we flew into all these canyons and checked out the volcanoes. This island is incredible.'

The same day, we packed a van, drank French beer and endeavoured a swim at the famous waterfalls called Trois Bassins. Quite simply, it means three basins in French. Amazingly, it is a series of waterfalls that cascade down a gorge into one big rock pool, then another, then another. It is beautiful. It was then, once we started driving around meeting people and watching the volcanic activity above us, that we discovered Reunion. The people there are a pretty even mix of African and French blood. French supermarkets like Le Clerc mix with island-style bars and French money. We learned that it was here that the first euro changed hands — because of the time difference with Europe — when their president bought a bucket of lychees from the local market. Reunion has that unique combination of European money and flair, plus the natural wealth of divine forests.

Reunion is home to one of the world's most active volcanoes — Piton de la Fournaise — which has erupted more than 170 times since the mid-seventeenth century. Lava flows have closed the roads, damaged buildings and put on shows for tourists on a daily basis; they have even built most of the reef breaks we surfed. There isn't much Reunion lacks at sea level, with epic waves and beautiful water that offers diving and surfing at world-class levels.

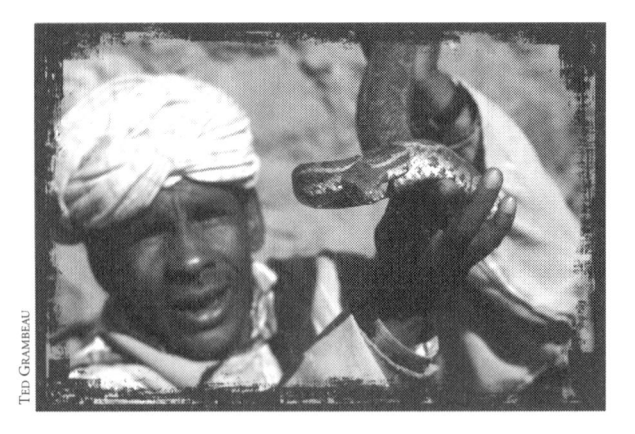

# LIVING THE MIRAGE
## MOROCCO

'Why are you going to Morocco now?' asked Manu, the Rip Curl licensee in Casablanca. 'It's Ramadan. Nobody has sex, alcohol, food or anything in daylight hours for one month.' I was in France planning my trip to Morocco and I thought I was starting to figure the place out. I was so wrong ...

I had arrived in Marrakech just before midnight and caught a taxi to an open-air hotel Manu had recommended. It was getting late — and the hotel was hard to find between the labyrinths of clay walls. The taxi parked next to a group of camels and donkeys, while kids played soccer on the pavement under breaking streetlights. A white foreigner carrying his surfboards towards the hotel completed the circus. But the locals didn't bat an eyelid. They were still packing their fruits, spices and snakes from the day's market.

The Arabic hotel name translated into something to do with Angels. The owner/operator was a rare Moroccan hippy, obviously into angels and seemed so high she may have had wings and been an angel herself. Or maybe it was the faint smell of hash that suggested a defied sense of gravity. Old Persian rugs lined the floor of this old structure, big smoking pipes — hookahs — lined the common living room and chanting could be heard from the big mosque down the road, where devout Muslims practised their faith.

'It is the big month of Ramadan,' the lady said. 'For one month we practise abstinence — refraining from the indulgences of the physical world and pray to Allah. It's good for the belly,' she said (the faithful don't eat during daylight hours), as her hand made circles on her middle-aged stomach. 'And good to stop drinking the alcohol,' she added, looking at the two tourists who straggled and stumbled towards their room. Between this town, the tourists, the history and the hash, there hasn't been much that this lady hasn't seen. From her hash-inspired height, she has had a good, if not interesting and calm view.

It was all a bit much to take in at that time of night when I had just arrived, so, in a cloud of smoke, I retired to my room as thoughts of Indiana Jones, snake charmers and the world's biggest open-air market joined my dreams.

## CHARMING SNAKES AND LADDERS

I awoke to the dawn session of chanting at the local mosque. Had the chanting ever actually stopped? The sun was starting to paint orange on the lower part of the horizon and slowly it lit up the city. The Arabs, who have occupied this land for as long as written history, tinkered with their produce, which was mainly spices, and packed their donkeys for the ride to the market.

Marrakech is called the 'Red City' because it is veneered with red mud and clay bricks. This gives it an organic feel and even in the most crowded part of the city, the red dust reminds you that this city is somewhat connected with an ancient world. Or, at least, combined with the dirt roads and donkeys, it reminds you it is in the Third World. The population of this place is just over one million, but you will see many more donkeys than cars.

The streets were alive with colours and fragrances: the smell of spices invaded my nostrils as I approached the massive market. It was early, and Moroccan men were setting up stalls that would sell the renowned orange juice, spices, dates, ceramics, silverware, carpets and artwork. The women were either at home, or dutifully on their way home. Veiled in black dresses that covered them from head to toe, they moved without making eye contact. It is forbidden by law. In this country, women are considered to be property owned by their husbands, who are the only ones who have the right to see their flesh. Their flowing dresses may have covered up all but their eyes, but they wore CK sunglasses as their window to the outside world — as if the last part of their bodies over which they had control was enjoying one small freedom.

The markets were enormous, as big as a small town itself, and you could easily get lost in the maze of colours and spices. I escaped for some famous mint tea and prepared for my meeting with the snake charmers. I'm not scared of snakes, but there's something freaky about touching them — or, even freakier, when they touch you. The charmers mock them, slap them on the head and watch them dance to the music of their flutes, safe in the knowledge that their fangs have been cruelly cut out — something that shouldn't sit well with the tourists who contribute to this performance. I approached them. When I say them, picture a cement plaza of about 200 metres square, fill it with around a hundred snake charmers and their flutes and snakes. The sound of the flutes can't soothe the noise of these hawkers demanding your attention and money. They compete for it, hawking and spruiking, and performing seemingly death-defying tricks with their snakes. Their mastery of languages and tricks is obviously spurred on by a sad desperation for something we have that they don't — money.

I sat down with one and soon the thrill and fear of the snakes — four of them — slithering all over my arms, legs and shoulders brought me back to the moment. It was very weird, but an experience you have to have if you go there. I'm sure Alexander the Great did it.

Marrakech was an interesting place, a mingling circus of humans and history — but it was full on! Soon, it was time to get back to salt water and adjust the pH levels. But there was something standing in the way.

## THE SAHARA

Picture endless sand. Infinite is a hard world for us humans, with our preoccupation for measuring things, to comprehend. But when you look over the Sahara Desert, it is like the infinity of space. Unforgiving rolling dunes are broken up by rocks that dot the sand like stars in the endlessness of space. It doesn't rain here, but the winds have made patterns in the few dunes that aren't covered by relentless rock. The drive was beautiful. Our driver was swift over the plains and cautious over the hills, whose blind corners often hid approaching donkeys. Even on the highway, donkeys are still the main form of transport for the Arabs.

Finally, we landed at a lookout and shared conversation with a couple of wind surfers. 'The wind is strong. Good for wind surfing and kite surfing but maybe not surfing, yes?'

They were glad to see some foreign surfers, as they wouldn't see many. Upon a dusty hilltop, we looked over the coastline, where the desert met the sea. The wind swept over the sand and the sea, creating arid waves on both. The sign in Arabic pointed us in the direction of the coast. I knew that much. We pulled out past a pack of camels and started for the ocean.

## LAND OF LONG RIGHT POINTS

Yann Martin is the European surf manager for Oakley Europe. A competitive surfer, he has three French titles — and a Moroccan passport — to his name. Though he has been living, competing and working in France for a while, Yann's roots run a little further south.

'I was born in Morocco and stayed there until I was nineteen,' said Yann. 'I started surfing there when I was ten. I went to school there and my whole childhood and teenage years were spent there. My mum was a teacher and my father was working for the King.'

Morocco is still a monarchical system, its servants ruled by the commandments of their King and their God. Yann was able to experience it all. He did a stint in the French Army, but found his way back to the ocean pretty fast. 'After the army I stayed in France and since then I go back to Morocco every year.'

I'd bumped into Yann in France, and as we were checking the surf we spoke about surfing in Morocco.

'Nobody used to surf there at all,' he said, looking over the coast. 'It's a little crowded now. More and more tourists are coming and more locals are starting to learn. But for the most part, all the guys have remained the same. They are super cool and like to talk with tourists. You know Moroccan hospitality is pretty famous.'

I have to say, the hospitality he talks about is definitely there. They have such a colourful and vibrant culture, and the opportunity to talk to a foreigner just adds more colour to their day, so they are very friendly and welcoming. They speak most languages starting with their own — Arabic — but French and English are also common. Even the French, who have as great an appreciation of culture as of wine, sometimes find the Moroccan way of life a little too spicy. It is completely different — and the fundamental difference starts with their religion.

'The Moroccan boys live with Allah [God] and that makes everything different,' explained Yann.

They live by different laws and go to the mosque all the time.

'I could talk for ten days about Morocco. But just one thing — you guys must go there to see that beautiful country, the people who live there, the places and the sun,' he finished.

## FRENCH FOREIGN REGION

In the late nineteenth century, European countries were setting sail and land grabbing all around the world, looking for natural resources and riches. It was the time of colonialisation, which led to races and wars — and wars between races. France, Spain and Germany made moves to hijack Morocco due to its strategic position and rich trade resources. France won and occupied virtually the entire country by 1912. But they didn't change too much — they probably couldn't. The same Arab people have lived here for as long as recorded history. It's what makes the culture so entrenched, unique and rich. Some of the country's businesses, schools and other institutions are still French, but they exist on rented land owned by history.

Eventually, independence secured Moroccan freedom in 1956. However, the locals speak with a French and Arabic tongue and many French remain, including our host for the next couple of days. He was a mild-mannered man of the world, who was embarking on a journey of epic proportions.

## MANU

Manu and his wife Estere have made Morocco their home for quite a few years. They are charged with the responsibility of building the Rip Curl brand in Africa. They will set up the flagship businesses in Morocco first, before moving to Madagascar or Senegal. They haven't decided yet, but there is a glimmer in their eyes at the thought of chasing new horizons. There is a little bit of the hippy/travelling surfer still flowing in both of their veins.

'We have a good life here. We can afford a really good house, a nanny for our baby, a good school … In Morocco we can live like kings on our European wage. We just couldn't do that in France anymore. We worked harder and harder — and were just getting by. The cities are so expensive and the lifestyle is so rushed. We are forgetting about the importance of lifestyle in Western society more and more, so we came here for that.'

Manu picked us up in his four-wheel drive and took us straight to check the surf near his home on the outskirts of Casablanca. It was a left. Can you believe it? I'd come all this way to see the famous right points and I was looking at a fat left. I shouldn't be so harsh. It was actually pretty good — as long as Raglan and, though a little flat, very rippable.

After close examination, Manu decided it would be better with the lower tide, so we headed back to his house for tea. His house was a miniature castle on a block of land so big you'd describe it as grounds. It was colourful and exotic, an open plan on open land, built with an open mind. The grass was manicured green and the flowers completed the oasis on this barren and dusty land, where just outside his gates, plastic bags blew like tumbleweed in the wind amongst other rubbish and dust. From the roof, you could see Casablanca off in the distance, a few big buildings with a blanket of city haze. The left we had just checked was in the valley below us, the first of many points in between here and the city.

The maid had his baby strapped to her back while she tinkered with dinner in the open kitchen. We sat in the courtyard and talked.

'Rip Curl is the only surf company here. Before us, the only way people here could get surf gear was if tourists left it as gifts. Usually, like in Indo, they would leave broken boards for them to fix and learn the art of riding waves — and fixing boards. It's an expensive process to get the boards here, and we basically sell them at cost price, just to get them out there.'

'How much is that?' I asked.

'Five hundred euros. That's the problem. The average monthly income here is two hundred euros, so they just can't afford it. It's a challenge.'

We were on our way to check the surf. A big southerly had found its way up the coast — and my dreams of surfing the infamous right-hand points were gone with the wind. Even though the land was hot, the water was cold due to the cold Atlantic currents.

We surfed for a few hours until our legs and arms gave out. Along with the surrounding desert and the setting sun, the ocean also reflected the orange, giving in to its glow and sinking into darkness.

When we came in we discovered an argument was going on between two local Moroccan surfers. Obviously they were talking in Arabic, so we understood nothing, but Manu, who is becoming fluent in the language, overheard them and went over to cool down the situation. He had just been saying how mellow the place was, and was disappointed and a little embarrassed by this display. 'It's the end of the month. Everyone has done twenty-eight days of Ramadan and they are getting agitated,' he said. 'People literally start going crazy. They drive faster. There are more crashes because they are frustrated without food, sex and alcohol. Anyway, I told them I had guests from Australia and they were bringing shame to our country. They stopped immediately and apologised. To put shame on your country is one of the worst possible things you can do here.'

That night we sat down for a traditional Moroccan meal with Manu, his family, and a friend of his, a former bodyboarding champion from France. As we sipped the local alcoholic mix, Manu showed us photos of the waves down south, in particular Anchor Point in Agadir, and Sufi. It only breaks four or five times a year, but the waves were so good, you'd convert to Islam just to sample one of them. It truly is one of the best waves in the world — an oasis in the Moroccan desert.

'We go on camping trips all the time. And not just for the waves,' said Manu. He showed me pictures of him and his wife standing in the massive caves in the beach. It looked beautiful, and the smiles on their faces proved it. Just before dinner was served — an oven-baked brew of meat, lentils and apricots in the traditional crockery pot called a tangine — we had to go down the street to get some bread. We had already heard the chanting from a nearby house, its volume turned up by Ramadan. But as we neared the shops, the sound of it was overwhelming.

'During Ramadan, they go to church five times a day — and pretty much repeat this at all times a year. The culture and religion here is bad,' said Manu. 'They can't drink according to the Koran. But there is nothing in the Koran about hash, ecstasy or cocaine, so the teenagers all release themselves on that. The law is ancient, you know — and the times change. There are few freedoms, especially for women.'

Make no mistake, here in Arabic/Muslim Morocco, the Koran is law. Manu's friend had fallen in love with a Moroccan girl, and asked for her hand in marriage. He explained the situation.

'If you are not from here, it would seem bad. But anyway, when you get a wife here, you have to buy her. Then she is yours — you literally own her. Muslim law dictates that I buy her from her father and convert to Islam. I loved her, so I had to do it.'

We finished our dinner and indulged in some Moroccan hash — and let the feeling of Morocco take over our thoughts.

## MOSQUE RIGHT

According to Manu, Casablanca is 'the economic capital of Africa'. With a population of six million, the whole place is growing, fertilised by the constant sprinkle of foreign investment. It's pretty weird to drive past donkeys and sand dunes one minute, and then big malls and chain stores like Starbucks and McDonald's the next. 'So many people are investing in Morocco now,' said Manu. 'New franchises, new big businesses. It's one of the fastest growing economies in the world.'

We checked some surf spots on the way and there were some outside ledges that showed a plethora of promise. The swell was big, around six to eight feet, but the strong south wind persisted and bumped up the face of what looked like amazing waves. 'What about that wave?' I asked.

'I don't think anyone has surfed that one. Maybe some bodyboarders?' You've got to remember, there are so few surfers here. And the ones who do surf — like Manu — aren't at a level where they can surf ledges. He actually rides a Malibu mostly. Opportunity lurked at the rise of every reef. I thought of Yann and how many lone surfs he would have had growing up here, of how good it would be to have a few months and go exploring, of finding new spots, surfing them, and naming them.

My head drifted with the idea and my eyes didn't even need to close to see the dream. Then a new scene stole my attention. At the end of a point overlooking the sea, the world's second biggest mosque rose from the ocean and extended to the heavens. It stood proudly taller than the surrounding capitalist buildings, an enormous structure that seemed to exist through divine intervention. I stood there watching it for a while — and the right-hander that broke off the breakwall built to protect it. Manu read my mind and intervened. 'You wouldn't be allowed to surf there, I don't think,' said Manu. 'Or at least it would be a little disrespectful, especially during Ramadan.' I looked at the guards, listened to the sound of chanting and let it overwhelm the thought of the waves.

## THE NEW GUARD

Abdel El Harim is the best surfer Morocco has ever had. He grew up in Rabat, the 'capitale of Morocco', where indulgences in the physical world are met with religious resistance, and the escapism involved with surfing contrasts the centre of their religion. Abdel was trying to find balance between the culture of the Koran and the freedom of the ocean.

'My brother is a surfer and he taught me how to surf. It was very difficult in the beginning because there was no surf shop here in Morocco. Nothing at all! We just bought secondhand material from the Oz, European and American surfers who came here. Seriously, the waves are perfect! We have every kind of wave here: reef barrels, beach breaks, long point breaks — and at any time of the year. But the south of Morocco needs so much swell to have good waves. The north, from Casablanca to Kenitra Mehdia beach, you can surf every day.'

Abdel became opportunistic and learned fast, borrowing boards, and then buying boards from travellers. Soon he became a pro, but the path of resistance was still there.

'When people see us go surfing in the winter they say, "You guys are crazy to go swim in the cold weather." But it's hard to be a pro surfer in Morocco. Firstly, the family wants you to do studies only, or to surf only on the weekend. Second, there's no money to buy surfing material, and third, you need a visa for everywhere to travel. It is very difficult to get this if you come from Morocco. You need a sponsor to send you papers to say that you're going to stay with a team and all kinds of stuff. This is one of the reasons I have never been to Oz. I have to go to Igipte [Egypt] just to get this visa, because we don't have an Australian Embassy in Morocco. But since 2007 we have had a federation of surfing, so the federation gives some surfing material to the top sixteen surfers and bodyboarders, which helps us travel.'

We talked about culture, about us all sharing the same dream of surfing, of riding waves to escape, but the details of the life of a Moroccan surfer were interesting to us.

'I don't know if it is like this everywhere in the world — you have good people and bad people,' said Abdel. 'People are cool here because they always try to help you. We are the only Muslim country in the world that doesn't have problems, so it says something about the place. We have a lot of different religions here because we have people from France, Spain and the United States living here. We have acceptance because we live with different ideas and don't fight them. I surf, but my life is different. I wake up at 6 am to pray in the mosque. I then go to the gym for training. I then pray again at lunch, go surfing and hang out with some friends. Then I pray again before dinner and go to sleep early.'

The surfing dream in Morocco is a little hard to realise, but with the help of Manu and the creation of a surf industry, plus a bit of social acceptance, things are on the move.

'If the new young Moroccan surfers get sponsored, surfing in Morocco will go far,' said Abdel. 'There are only four surfers with a sponsor here in Morocco — three juniors and me. I'm twenty-two years old now and I do everything I can to get into the World Tour. Like we say at home — "If God wants."'

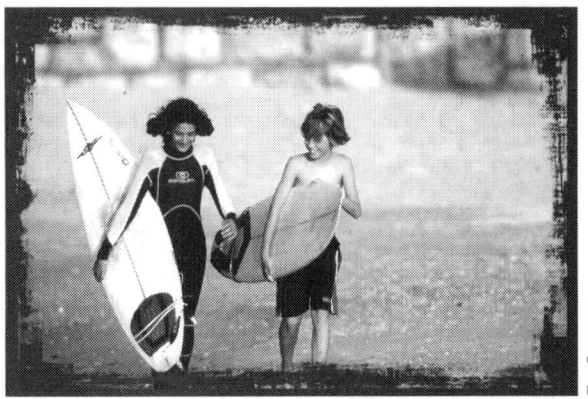

# THE LONG WALK
## ISRAEL

Above and beyond more real estate, this piece of 'holy land' is the centre of everything good and bad in the world. It's the 'Promised Land' to the Jewish community, and struggle and persecution have been taking place for years over the historic dust where God first sang the Ten Commandments. It may not have beaches like J-Bay, Pipeline or Kirra, but it has places like Jerusalem, Bethlehem and Mount Sinai. Israel may have no famous surfing names like Kelly Slater, Mick Fanning or Joel Parkinson, but Jesus, Abraham and Moses lived and taught in this ancient place. Wars have been fought, lands have been returned, waters have been parted, commandments have been given. And all the while, waves have greeted her shores — legitimate waves with passionate followers as committed to their wave riding as their religion. Israel is a place that will surely swell the soul and its antiquity stirs something even deeper.

# TEL AVIV

There I was, checking the surf on a beach just north of Tel Aviv. How strange! Outside, the afternoon air cooked my shoulders as I regarded the waves below the small sandstone cliff with surprising enthusiasm. It was two to three feet, and little peaks stirred the shallow sand bank, rising up with creativity. I was in the far southeast corner of the Mediterranean Sea looking at legitimate waves in a land best known for other mysteries.

Around twenty to thirty surfers rode the waves while even more were coming and going, commuting, like the rush of peak hour in a city of sand and salt. 'Surfing is huge here,' said Yossi Zamir, my good friend from Australia who grew up here. Yossi, now thirty-one, has lived in Australia for twelve years now. He owns a bar at Bondi Beach — Bunga Bar — but makes the trip back to Israel at least once a year to reconnect with his roots. He was the one who talked me into the trip and he had started day one with purpose.

'When there are waves here, people drop everything and go surfing,' said Yossi, looking up and down his beach of origin as if he was looking at a photo album. He was excited by the two-foot waves. 'It's not like Australia here. In Israel, if it's breaking, there are waves. It doesn't get over four feet very often. And when it does, you have to move. I've heard of people leaving their pregnant wives in hospital to go surf!'

Yossi, like most Israelis, loves the beach and was one of the first generation of surfers to get any good at the sport. Entering the water, he gave a wave to his friends who all paddled over to return the respect, and meet his foreign friend. The water provided little relief from the heat as the temperature was above 30 degrees Celsius. The ocean was like a bath, but between the sea breeze, the hospitality of the people and the ocean, I was inspired for my first surf in Israel.

The hospitality there is truly amazing. The people were all stoked to meet a foreigner, talk surf stories and share their waves and thoughts. You could tell that not many of them would ever have the chance to leave Israel, so meeting a foreigner was the next best thing. We rode waves for an hour before Yossi took me to one of the many bars on the beach for a beer.

## THE PROMISED LAND

I was on the beach, having a beer and listening to the sound of the waves mixed with the sound of fresh European DJ vibes. The sun was sinking over the sea, the orange sky reflecting its warmth on the water. A very Westernised crowd — influenced by the many tourists from France, Russia, Spain and Portugal — gathered in the bars. And of course there were beautiful women everywhere. It could have been Ibiza. The locals — well, the locals have a story to tell indeed and over a beer Yossi gave me a summary of the evolution of the Jews. (This was not told to me by God himself, and since I'm not endeavouring to rewrite the Bible, please excuse any inaccuracies in his modest appraisal.)

'It started when Moses first marched the Jews back from Egypt, freeing them from slavery and taking them to the "Promised Land".'

'How long ago was that?' I asked.

'Fuck, man, that's back in the Bible. I don't know, maybe five thousand years?'

But the story started much earlier — with a bloke named Abraham. Yossi continued.

'He was the first Jewish person. When he was 100 or something God gave him a present — a son — just before he died. His name was Isaac. Now, God asked for this son to be sacrificed and when Abraham went to do it, God, impressed by his commitment, stopped him and said, "Save your son. If you really believe me, I promise you the Jewish nation — and you will have the same amount of followers as there are stars in the sky." Or the sand on the beach — something like this. Anyway, Abraham had two sons — Isaac and Ishmael — and Isaac also had two kids, Jacob and Esau. These two brothers had a big fight and that's when the faith split. One of them — Esau — went east into the desert, where the seeds of the Muslim religion would soon dig in their roots.

'When he was in Egypt, Joseph had a dream about seven fat cows, which was followed by a dream about seven skinny cows. He saw this as a symbol of seven abundant years for Egypt, followed by seven lean years. Somebody told the pharaoh, who believed in this sort of thing and took Joseph's word for it. The pharaoh stored food and prepared for seven bad years of hardship and, by doing this, basically saved Egypt because Joseph's vision came true. So Joseph became an important and powerful man in Egypt.

'As he thought the Jews were then starting to gain too much power in Egypt, the pharaoh concocted a plan to kill all the first-born Jewish boys to stop the spread of Jewish influence. A woman had a baby called Moses; to protect him from certain death, she put him in a basket of reeds and let the river hide him.

'Someone found Moses and raised him, and when he came to power, he demanded that the people be let free. The Egyptians refused and God punished them. One of the ten punishments was that all the liquid in Egypt turned to blood. The last punishment was the killing of all the oldest boys in every Egyptian family in one night.

'Then all the Jews left with Moses for the promised land. God had promised it. When they reached the Red Sea, Moses parted the sea and the Jewish people went through, while God closed the waters on the Egyptians and they died.

'So they reached Mount Sinai and that's where God gave song to the Ten Commandments and reality to the "Promised Land".'

There was no evidence of any interruption of the Jewish occupation of this land for the next three millennia. Then people started warring over land and religion — and Zion, or Palestine as it would later be known — was the prize. On this land is the world's first church — Solomon's Temple, which was built by King Solomon. It was the birthplace of the Old and New Testaments, the place where the Ten Commandments were spoken from a bush of fire and where three wise men found baby Jesus and where he was crucified and rose from the dead. It is also believed to be the place of creation, where God made the first rock — and ultimately the world. All right here, under the temple mount. The Romans eventually burnt down Solomon's Temple, leaving only one wall intact — the West Wall. Palestine — the place where modern religion was born — was becoming the most hostile place on earth.

'It's all over the land,' said Yossi. 'All the Arab countries want Jerusalem, but we don't want to give it up. It's stupid because it all comes from the same God anyway. The only difference is the one brother who taught something a little different.'

The land was fought over, the Jews were forced to flee time and time again, and for generations the universal theme of the ingathering of the exiles and the re-establishment of the kingdom of Israel carried predominantly religious overtones. This was due to the belief that the Jewish people would return to Zion with the coming of the Messiah, that is, after divine intervention. The Jews moved around the world trying to find peace while waiting for that divine intervention. But Europe and Arabia decided they didn't like the Jewish people anymore and anti-Semitism flared like fire, even before Hitler killed six million Jews in the Nazi Holocaust of the last century. The Jews had no home.

'Why did they get such a hard time?' I asked. Yossi explained: 'Basically, no one likes people who are different; they fear difference. So firstly they were disliked because they look different; they wear black and the *kippahs* [the small cap worn to give respect and distance between heaven and earth] on the head and stuff like this. Second, they were always very successful people. They always had money, and were controlling this and that. I think that was the core of anti-Semitism. In Germany, they threw all the Jews out of their jobs and then killed them. It was the same in Spain. They didn't let the Jews study anything but their version of Catholicism, and when Jews studied their own religion secretly, the Spanish started persecuting them and hanging them.'

Napoleon once said that history is written by the winners of war — and I was starting to believe the same thing of the Bible.

While they waited in exile, some Jewish leaders proposed a return, but they were in a minority. Then they slowly came back, waiting for their true messiah. 'Jesus was a Jew,' said Yossi. 'But we didn't believe he was the Messiah. That's the difference between Jews and Christians. So again, it's the same God but a few different details — and that's what all the fighting has always been about.'

The fighting over the land — because it is a holy place to Jews, Christians *and* Muslims — continued until 14 May 1948 when the state of Israel was created.

'The Jews had their home and it didn't matter where you were from — if you were a Jew, you were in.' But the troubles didn't stop there ...

## SURFING IS MY RELIGION

Rising at our back, the sun was beginning to light the Mediterranean. The waves were two feet — again. Not quite enough to leave your wife in hospital with your first child, but probably enough to take the day off school or work. The busy car park confirmed my thoughts. The wind swells dumped their momentum on the shallow sand bank, waiting for the afternoon wind to break them into peaks. There were already twenty people out — and more getting ready in the car park. The word was out: there were waves. Yossi and I surfed for an hour before having lunch with Artur Rashkovan, the editor of Israel's surfing magazine. Together, we spoke of surfing in Israel over plates of hummus, pickles and meat.

'Being an Israeli surfer is like being a fish out of water pretty much,' he said. 'Up until the early nineties, people didn't travel very much and were not aware of what was going on in the outside world of surfing. And because of that, people weren't aware of Israel. It's funny: when I go on surf trips people are surprised to see good surfers from Israel. People don't even know we have an ocean. So I get comments like "No way, aren't you supposed to ride camels or something?"

'I think that being a surfer in Israel is a very unique thing, appreciated especially at times of war. We all need to thank someone — I don't who — that we have an ocean and we received the gift of surfing as a source of the most pure joy on earth.'

Israeli surfing started in 1956 when Dorian Paskowitz, regarded as the oldest Jewish surfer at eighty-six, brought the first surfboard to Israel. 'Since then it has developed into a big industry,' said Artur, 'with six shapers, local fashion brands and reps from all the big surf brands in the world.

'In 1985, a surfing association was formed, holding six to ten contests a year, and in 1987 the national surf team came third in the European Surf Championships, which was their first appearance. The surf school industry is very successful here in Israel too and today I believe that we have about 25,000 surfers across the country and 400 kilometres of coast.'

The sport and the industry have exploded. But, like the land around them, the ocean was a desert of little opportunity. So they searched for greener pastures.

'For Israeli surfers the future is all about surf travel, travel and more travel — especially for those who want to become pros. They need to leave the country as soon as they can and go to Europe in order to participate in as many contests as they can.'

These days, you can see Israeli surfers all around the world. Often they are mistaken for Brazilians because they share the same passion and skin colour — and what Artur describes as 'a need to learn more about ethics in the water'. The standard is getting better — and some are taking Artur's direct advice and heading overseas to try and be the first successful professional Israeli surfer.

## LOOKING FOR GOLD

One surfer chasing the dream is Gil Zilca. At nineteen, Gil captures the passion of Israeli surfing with every early surf. He has a soft nature and build, but surfs all day every day in the Mediterranean slop, hardening his skills; he is passionate about his desire to improve and to surf professionally. There is no real money in surfing in Israel yet. Some forward-thinking companies are paying for the country's top pros to compete in Europe, but that's about the extent of the finances. To further his career, Gil moved to the Gold Coast where the points of Surfers Paradise seemed like heaven.

'The waves in Australia are so amazing,' he said, eyes lighting up. 'Oh my God! And the level of surfing is way beyond anything in Europe, let alone Israel, so it's really hard. I just go in the QCC (Queensland Championship Circuit) and do the Junior Series as well. I can't believe how many good surfers are in Australia. Here in Israel, I am one of the best, but on any day on the Gold Coast, there are thousands of people who surf amazingly. It's really good as it helps me to improve.'

Gil is coming thirty-seventh on the QCC ratings in Queensland and has made it through some heats in the Billabong Pro Teen Junior Series contests. 'But that's even harder,' he said. 'I just need to keep trying my hardest and continue learning.'

We surfed together one day with Yossi. His board talks and his body torques at the level of the average surfer on an Australian or American beach, and his surfing did command some respect in Israel. People knew who he was, they shared his dream. But the steps he needs to take for him to realise his dream may also undermine it. 'I know that to get better I have to live outside Israel. Here the waves aren't consistent enough and I need to be around good surfers. But at the moment, in Australia, the surfers are a lot better than me and it's hard to get waves.'

Gil married an Australian girl, making his stay in Oz smoother, but the path to professional surfing won't be as easy. However, time and passion are on his side. As we sat out the back talking all things surf with the other hopeful kids in the area, I learned that there is another reality in Israel that can arrest the personal aspirations of its surfing youth.

# SERVICE

At the age of eighteen, every Israeli youth must do military service. It reshapes their life in ways we cannot understand. Yossi also did his time. Talking with me, he reflected on his country's reasons for demanding this service, and on the personal consequences.

'Israel is a very small country, surrounded by several Arab countries [Egypt, Saudi Arabia, Jordan, Syria, Iraq and Lebanon] that want to destroy us. We have to be strong to defend ourselves. There are not enough people to have an army of volunteers, so military service has to be compulsory. We'd rather not have any but it's a heavy situation and something we grow up with in Israel.

'In one day you grow from a little boy into a full-on adult. After two days you've got a gun in your hand; you have responsibility. The way they run it is with orders; you need permission to do anything. You can go to jail for disobedience. It sounds tough, but when you're standing in front of things you would never normally have to deal with, it builds strength and character in you.

'Even girls! Once she turns eighteen, a girl is holding a gun too, learning how to use it, running for kilometres with all the army gear on her back. That's what we do! You do this for eighteen months straight with six hours a night sleep max. You learn first aid, dealing with major wounds, confrontation … Not many people like it when they are in it, but you appreciate it afterwards because it builds you as a person and you learn how to treat people equally. It doesn't matter what colour you are, how much money your parents have, if you're a Russian or Israeli Jew — you treat everyone the same way. That's what I took from the army.'

Time has cast a positive light over his experiences, but there were some tragedies that Yossi will never forget.

'We went with some of our team for a border check, maybe six or eight of us. We were in the middle of the desert and there was a Russian guy with us. Basically we were doing four hours' patrol, two hours' sleep, then four hours' patrol for two weeks straight. One day this Russian guy was supposed to wake me up and he didn't. I went to look for him and couldn't find him anywhere. I eventually found him against the wall of the generator. He had shot himself through the head. His blood and head were all over the wall.

'People died fighting, people died from accidents, people died from a lot of things. I saw a suicide bomber at a bus stop next to my house one time; he killed many of our friends.

'They're just kids, you know. They're only eighteen, nineteen, twenty, so it's sad to put them through this, but it's something Israel can't survive without. If we didn't have the military service, we wouldn't have a country.'

I asked him if he thought it would ever change.

'Things are getting better now,' Yossi replied. 'Things like surfing are bringing new ideas and freedom to the younger generation. They don't think about the struggles of the past anymore. Everyone has got internet so they are more aware of the outside world. The differences between Israel and the rest of the world are becoming smaller and smaller. The actual people want peace, but it's up to the government. Even now, a big agreement with the Palestinians is still being blocked.

'We want to surf everywhere, without problems. The trouble all started from religion but it's not just that anymore; it's all about the land. They [the Arabs] believe that Israel is their land. We gave Jordan, Egypt and Palestine — we gave so much land just because we want to have peace, but it's not enough. It's all about Jerusalem — and Israel will never give that away.'

## HEAVEN AND HELL

So there I was in Jerusalem. The 'Old City' as they call it, has been rebuilt eight times in its long war-torn history. Dig deep enough and you might find a pair of Jesus' sandals, or at least an Arabian camel stirrup. Built into the hills of the Israeli interior (around 50 kilometres from the coast), Jerusalem is the bellybutton of modern religion and no matter your origin of faith (which by the way is defined in at least one dictionary as 'a belief in something that doesn't exist'), the energy here will stir something in you.

You won't find a point break, but you will find Solomon's Temple, the world's first house of God. I watched people cry at her wall; Christians, Jews and Muslims all side by side praying to the same God, but reading from different bibles. This place has changed the lives of people. They kneel at the walls, write notes and stick them between the mortar next to other people who do the same. It is peaceful and powerful, poignant and persistent — and whether you believe or not, there's some antique energy here that stirs you. But it is harmonious, a contrast to the extremism we see on television — our only window to this part of the world. At the church, there were no suicide bombers, no fighting. I saw religion the way it was designed to be.

Between the desert canyons, twenty minutes out of Jerusalem, Yossi's car followed the valley, snaking like water — down ... and down some more. Ears were in constant equalisation mode and all senses readjusted to the decline. From the bottom of the world (380 metres below sea level), the Dead Sea is a huge valley separating two mountain ranges between Jordan and Israel. The water is receding at a rapid rate. What look like tide lines mark where the sea used to lap the shore in years past, the salt staining layers of sand for hundreds of metres, as if marking birthdays.

Hot gases rose in the air as if the devil himself was trapped behind the sand. The mineral-rich salt is said to be therapeutic and the feeling of floating in the Dead Sea was like no other experience. 'It's impossible to drown here,' said Yossi. After walking through the water I began to discover why: I was so buoyant in the water that it felt like I was walking on the moon — the forces of this weird nature pushing my body upwards constantly, defying gravity.

The day finished with a *kippah* on my head and a seat at the dinner table with Yossi's family. 'The food here is the best in the world,' said Yossi. And he would know. The meal consisted of a mix of many small plates: hummus and all sorts of pickled meats, spices, fruits and vegetables. Yossi's dad read from the Jewish Bible (more as a cultural tradition than a leap of faith), we drank from the same glass as a toast, and ate our meal with cultural deference.

## GAZA

Things between Palestine and Israel aren't so snug, and the land in limbo has been at the centre of much fighting, debating and bleeding for a long time. But on Tuesday, 21 August 2007, a small gesture from a surfer changed some hearts.

The father of Israeli surfing, Dorian Paskowitz, brought two surfboards as part of a personal donation to Palestinian youths in the Gaza Strip. It wasn't the first time the idea had been born. Four years earlier, Artur, who had directed the Israeli Surfing Association, was asked by Dorian to meet some Arab surfers.

'When we met together I came up with the idea of holding an Arab–Israeli contest,' said Artur. 'So I did and it was a great success. Two years later, Dorian arrived with some soft-top surfboards to teach the next generation to surf, and we really bonded. He mentioned how great it would be to take boards to Gaza. It sounded a bit far-fetched to me. But since the idea was just to provide them with a pure source of joy and not to make some kind of a political statement, we didn't give up.

'In July of that year, Dorian read in the *LA Times* about two surfers in Gaza, sharing one board, who surfed to forget the troubles of their life in the Gaza Strip. Dorian was actually in Israel already to organise a big event named Surfing for Peace.

'This is where our foundation of Surfing for Peace turned into a real deal. I organised fifteen boards from all the shapers of Israel, with the help of an organisation named 'One Voice' [www.onevoice.org]. They have a rep inside Gaza who knew the surfers and got them to wait for us at the other side of the border. So through him we delivered the boards and then we [Surfing for Peace] became the target of all the press. It was hysterical. I was on the phone and on email for seventy-two hours non-stop. But that's not the point. What I felt at that moment was that we were making a change, since our gesture was pure and from the people, to the same people on the other side — from a surfer to a surfer, no politics involved. Maybe this would be the beginning of a change.'

Since June 2007, when the armed militants of Hamas seized control of Gaza, Israel had kept the strip sealed off. Only essential and emergency supplies were allowed in. So when Dorian's helpers rolled up with fifteen surfboards to the fortified crossing, the guards put it bluntly: 'You can't go in.' But Dorian wouldn't take no for an answer.

Palestinian surfers were waiting on the other side so he made it clear to the guards that he had come thousands of kilometres — from the USA — to make this happen. In the end, they let them through.

Artur explained: 'What it means to me is very simple. I have a dream of surfing across the Mediterranean, and I know that these guys have the same dream. I hope that one day I'll be able to surf in Gaza. I can't go into Gaza right now, but maybe one day I will. I'm saying something very basic. Maybe we have conflicts between us, but the argument is over the land not the water so let's go out together and forget about it for a second.' Dorian has a saying: 'God will surf with the devil if the waves are good'.

'I believe the guys that got the boards have a new target ahead of them — to share the joy of surfing with their people and I know they will cherish what we did for the rest of their lives. This is just the beginning, though. We are going to support them with all the knowledge and experience we have gained through the years; teaching surfing, shaping, ding repair, contests etc. Next week I'm meeting the two guys and they will join me for a full day in Tel Aviv. To me we are just surfers. I don't care about nationalities and religion. Surfing is my religion.'

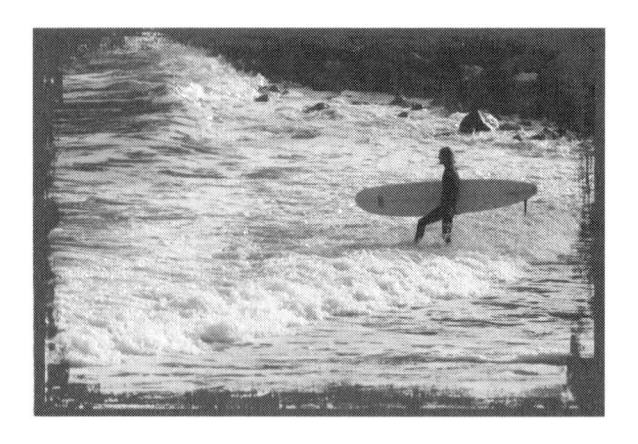

# BENEATH A MONOTONE SKY
## ENGLAND

In a seaside town called Plymouth on the south coast of England, a new day was beginning. As it was summer, the sun had come up early, but as we were in England, it was behind about seventeen layers of cloud. The clouds weren't fluffy and they didn't take any particular shape. They weren't black with hard rain, or broken by bits of blue or glowing orange from the sunrise; the sky was just a shapeless and colourless grey. People were going about their business. Their day starts with a cup of tea, backed by a cooked breakfast of sausages, eggs, baked beans and toast. People peered out the windows constantly, never giving up hope, always watching the weather — waiting. Massive seagulls complained about the lack of activity in the fish and chip shop that was yet to open; mechanical street cleaners washed the roads of the previous night's festivities.

The university up the road had just become the first university in the world to teach surfing as a subject, and so surfers had come. You could see the posters in the cafes, the stickers on the Kombi wagons, the occupants of which were busy trying to find the day's waves to wash off their hangovers. Out on the little island off the point, an old fortress told stories of war. Some of the stories are older than the Middle Ages. It was the weekend, the weather was still grey and everyone was participating in indoor activities: talking, tea-drinking, smoking and laughing. Doing what the English do.

Then the sun came out. All of a sudden, the streets were alive. People ran to the beach and to momentarily bake in the sun; mums were in the parks with their kids; people were happy. Then the sky turned to grey again and the people went back to their indoor activities, back to peering out the window, waiting. This lasted the rest of the day.

A game of soccer started, which led to beer-drinking. Since there are more pubs than corner stores, this is quite an easy pastime. Chelsea had just won against Manchester United. It was a big game and the Chelsea supporters looked over their pints of beer at the opposing supporters and started singing in practised unison, laughing and clapping: 'Look at the scoreboard.'

It's something England herself does every now and again — and so she should. She built the world's biggest empire, gave the world its global language, conceptualised most of the world's law, gave birth to industrialisation, became home to the world's first parliamentary democracy and developed most of the world's art, music and humour. All from a tiny place with a massive population (fifty-one million). Beneath a monotone sky, there is plenty of colour in English life — and it shows in many more places than Plymouth.

The plane was in a holding pattern. We had arrived early, so the 747 was doing circles, waiting for the end of the curfew that would allow us to land. Outside the window, there were at least twelve planes doing the same thing at different altitudes. There were layers of planes like layers of clouds. It would take more than the shapeless grey to upset the methodical harmony of organising a plane a minute to land.

Cities are odd things. They congregate commerce, people and their habitat. Encompassing the complete spectrum of race, culture and wealth — or lack of it — you can see everything in London. Many people come to London to work, earn the pound and travel around continental Europe. As it has one of the world's busiest airports and is the nucleus of capitalism, lastminute.coms and other cheap websites offer ridiculous prices to the European mainland. London is the port of entry and exit for almost everywhere people want to go. Some people arrive in London and work for years straight. Chances are, you probably know one of them. They boast of how the Australian work ethic means it's easy to get a job; they talk of playing pool and throwing darts in pubs, of football and the royal family, geezers and whingers, artists and musicians. There's a lot to do in cities and London has it all. Some people, however, have little interest in big cities apart from people-watching, and prefer to go straight to the beach.

Newquay is about a four-hour drive from London. There are many surfers who live in London and undertake the drive on weekends to get into the salt and ride some waves. It's a pleasant journey, past rolling green hills, Stonehenge, properties with hedges for fences, old pubs and the odd castle. But it is hard work being a surfer in England. Nobody knows this better than the current editor of *Surf Europe*, Paul Evans.

Paul grew up in Crowthorne, Berkshire, near London and was first introduced to surfing when he lived in California when he was eleven.

When he moved back to Crowthorne, surfing was a little harder — for a lot of reasons.

'I used to get a ride to the coast [a three-hour drive] with a bisexual, older friend who wanted to fiddle with me in return for lifts. This happened until I was seventeen and got my licence,' Paul said.

I met Paul through a mutual friend and his stories always cracked me up. Paul eventually moved to Plymouth, where he studied at the university. Andy King, Kieren Perrow and I would squash onto couches and floors and drive to Newquay from there for the WQS event. Paul is a funny bastard, and he'd entertain us with stories about his first trips to the coast and of enduring homosexual advances to get to the surf. 'He'd try all the time. It was pretty funny. It was the only way I could get to the beach so I kind of played dumb.

'Needless to say, I was pretty keen then so it was get a lift with the gay dude or don't go. I wasn't really that suspicious that a guy of nineteen wanted to hang out with a fifteen year old. I just assumed I must have been pretty fucking cool for my age. Anyway, we didn't have money to stay in a B&B so we slept in the back of his Uno [a tiny car, even by European standards]. It was actually pretty heavy really. The guy had a lot of really really serious issues and used to try and kill himself all the time. Sometimes I'd come back from the surf and he wouldn't be there. I'd run up the cliffs and find him and we'd have these huge dramatic don't-do-its in the howling wind. In the middle of the night too — just in the middle of total nowhere in mid-winter Cornwall — he'd try and top himself and I'd have to talk him out of it in these raging southwest gales in the dark. He also used to black out a lot; just pass out and start making these crazy throat

a wave away [209]

noises. Every time before we went away I'd know exactly what would be coming. But I guess I must've figured it was a worthwhile hassle to be able to surf.

'Then I passed my driving test and my dad lent me his car one Tuesday. It took about three hours on the motorway to get to Croyde. I stopped for a piss by the side of the road in the North Devon hills. It was a glorious spring day; flowers in the hedgerows, lambs bleating up and down green hills and valleys. The waves were clean, fun and uncrowded. I got a drive-thru Big Mac meal in Barnstable, ate it flying back towards London and remember thinking to myself, "Fuck yeah."

'I didn't mind being so far from the coast because I just devoured *Surfer* magazine and imagined surfing perfect waves rather than being in the freezing brown slop in Cornwall. I saved up ten pounds a week from my paper round and bought one of Spencer Hargrave's [former pro from England] old boards in 1991 for £200 in Newquay.'

Perspective sometimes only comes through distance. Paul now lives in France where he edits *Surf Europe*. With few ties left to England, his views on the 'Mother Country' are changing.

'It's very hard to say what being English exactly means today, particularly since I haven't lived there since 2003. To me, I'd like to think it would always mean a sense of fair play, cricket. In reality, we're a crowded nation of overweight, unhealthy, debt-ridden rampant consumers headed towards moral and spiritual bankruptcy, despite the fact that economically our country is very strong. If there were still one redeeming trait, it would probably be that the English, or the Brits, have more of a tendency towards humour than anyone else, certainly in Europe. Otherwise, returning back there from time to time, it's difficult not to

Morocco

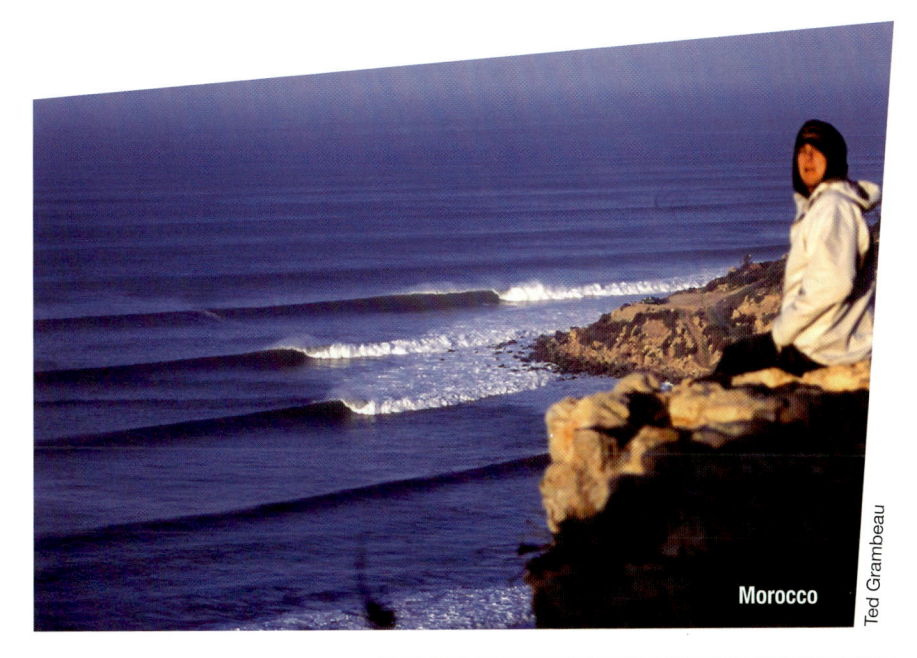

The ancient culture of Morocco has it all. From the perfect right-hand point breaks around Sufi (above) to the hustle and bustle of the world's largest open-air market in Marrakech (right). There are cultural, religious and geographical surprises around every corner.

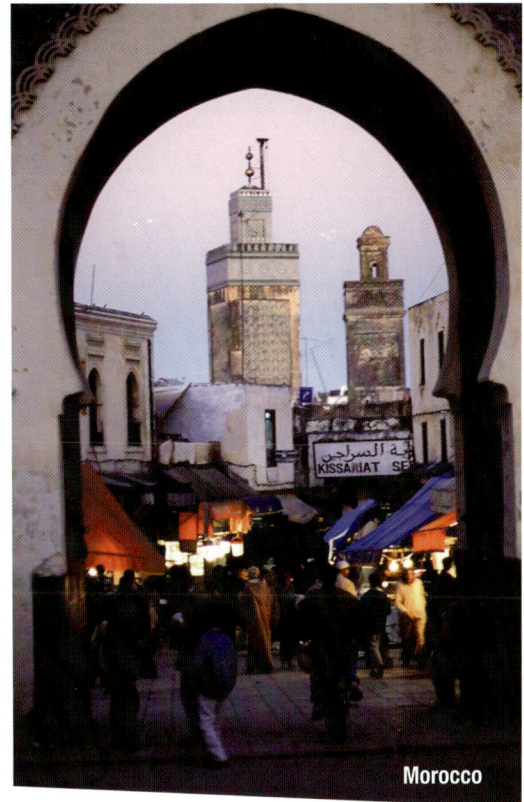

Morocco

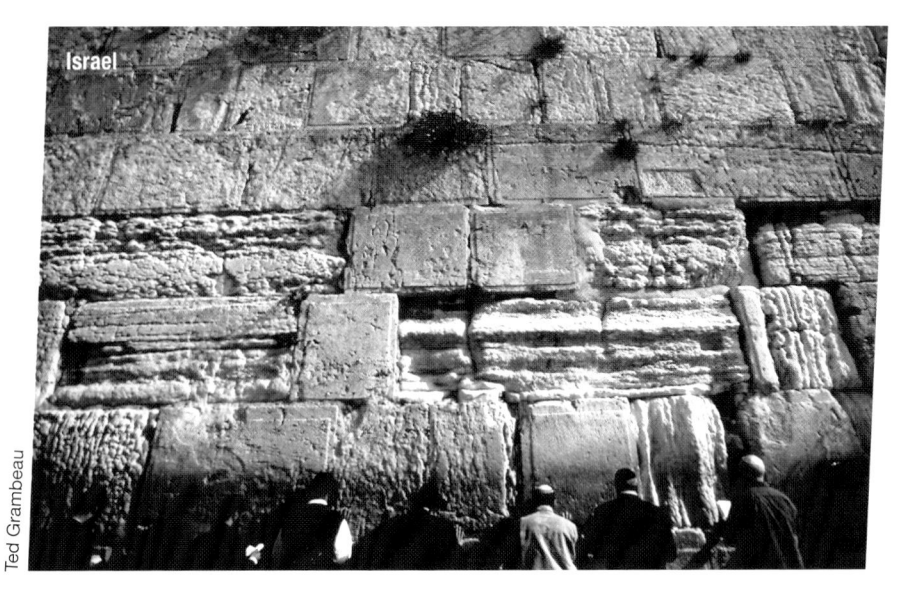

The west wall of Solomon's Temple (above) in Jerusalem. It is said by believers that the very first rock that started creation is below the temple: the world's first house of God. Only the west wall remains after several conquests. Here, some Jews pray at the wall, writing their prayers on pieces of paper and inserting them between the ancient stones. Whether you believe or not, the emotion can't help but stir the soul.

The shifting beach breaks around Tel Aviv (below) can get really fun. The nightlife, also mostly on the beaches, can be even more fun.

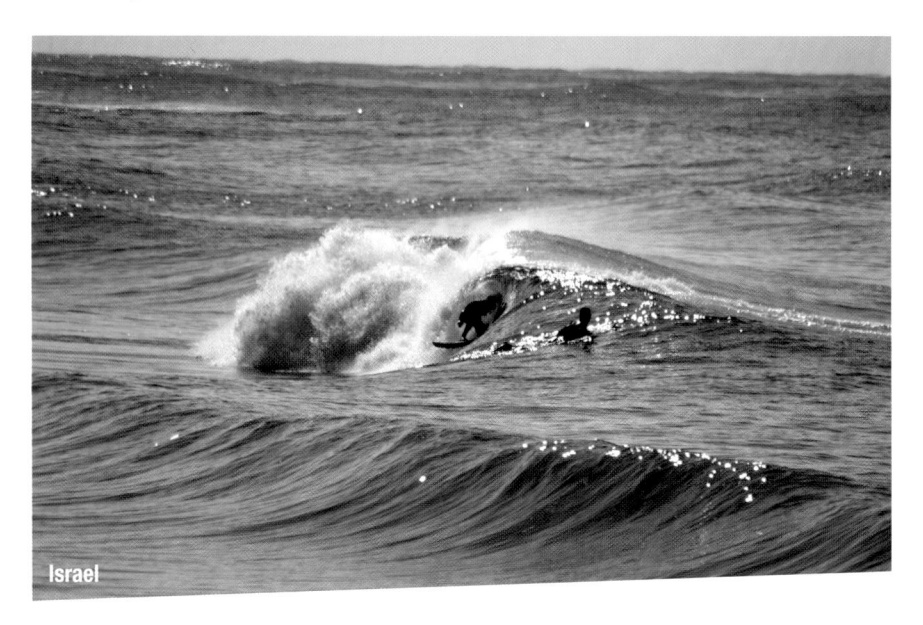

**Norway**

*Ted Grambeau*

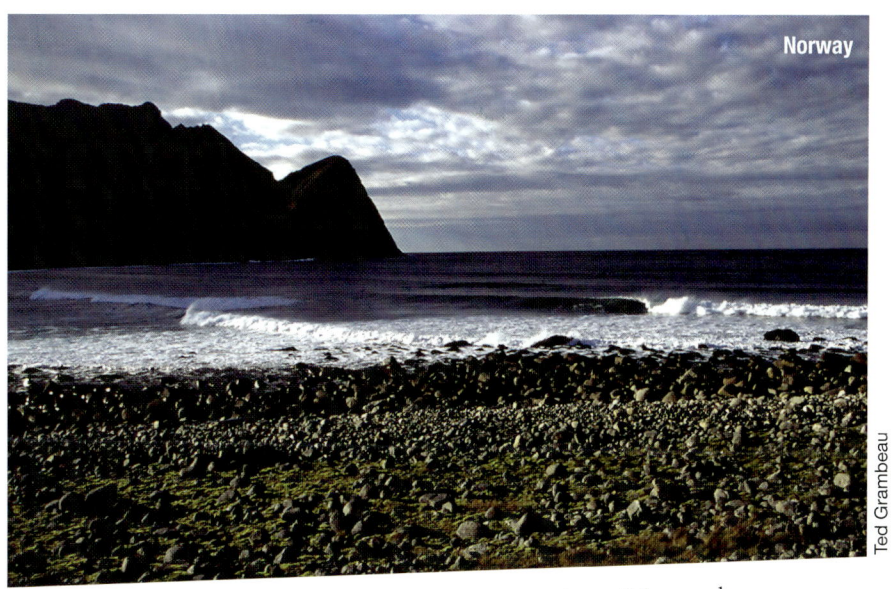

Cold water, big mountains and the voices of deceased Vikings whispering in the cold winds.

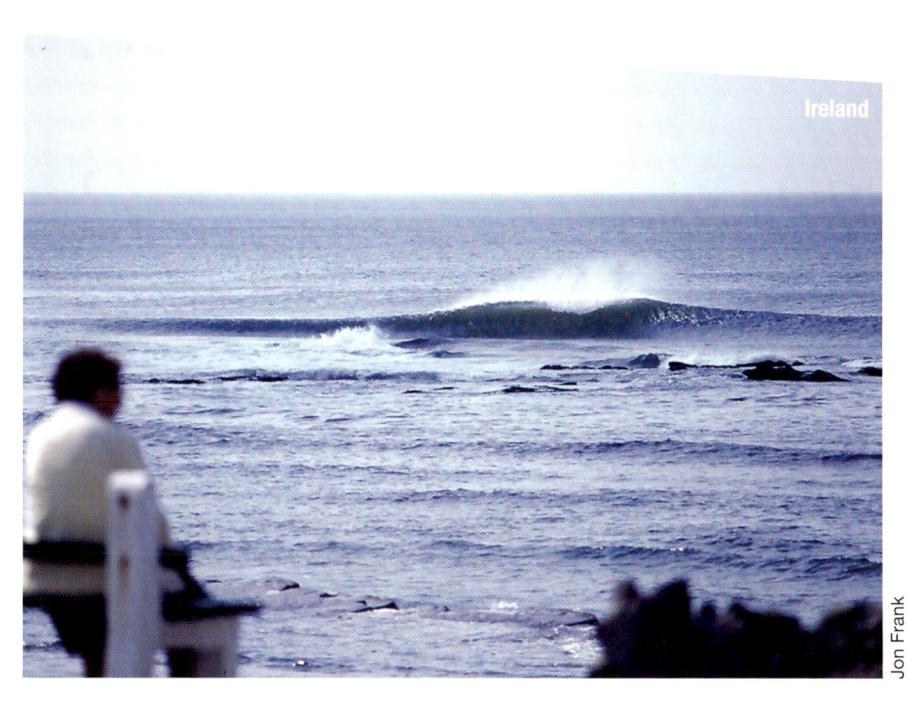

**Ireland**

*Jon Frank*

Ireland is littered with ledges and reef breaks, mostly unnoticed by the colourful locals. When the wind stops, Elysium is everywhere.

France

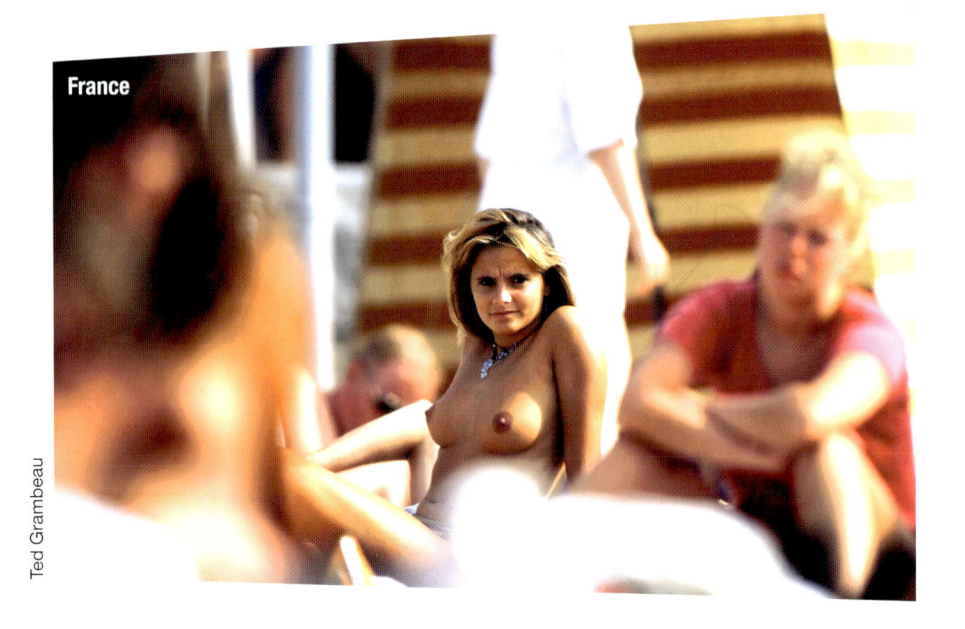

These two photos pretty much sum up the lure of France. But the culture offers so much more, making France the most visited place by tourists worldwide.

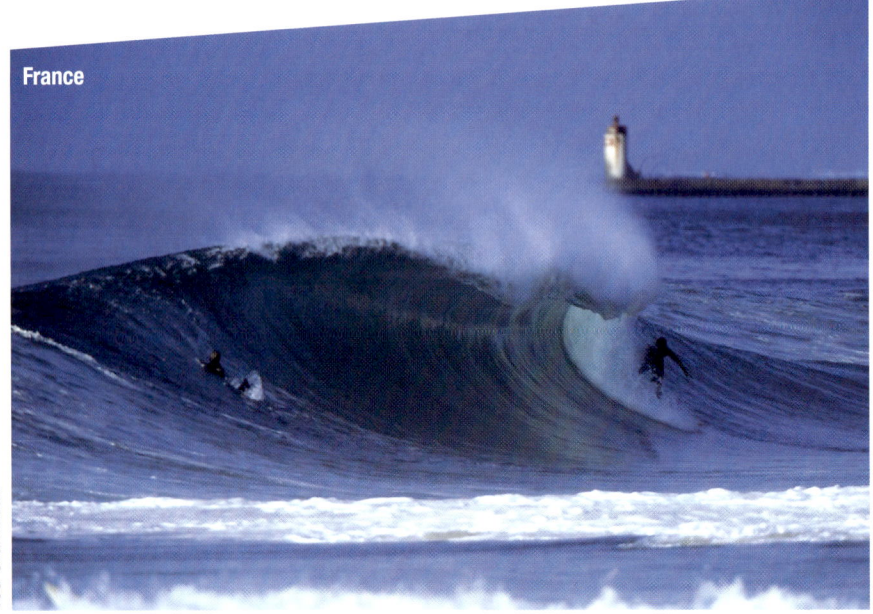

France

Ted Grambeau

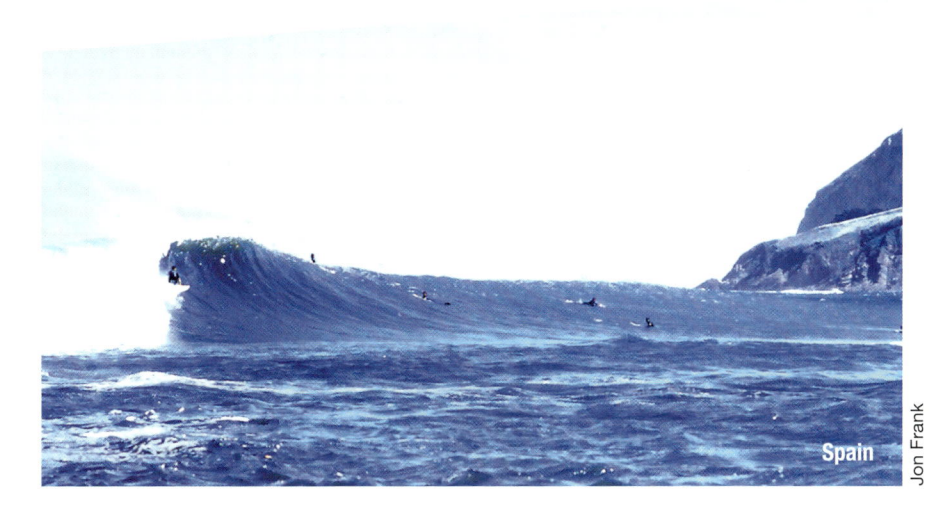

Mundaka (above) in the Basque country of Spain: it may not break all the time, but when it does, it could just be the best wave in the world. Medieval castles (below) show Spain's history and cultural diversity. This history collides with the independence-seeking Basque people who believe, 'Before there was God, there was the Basque country.'

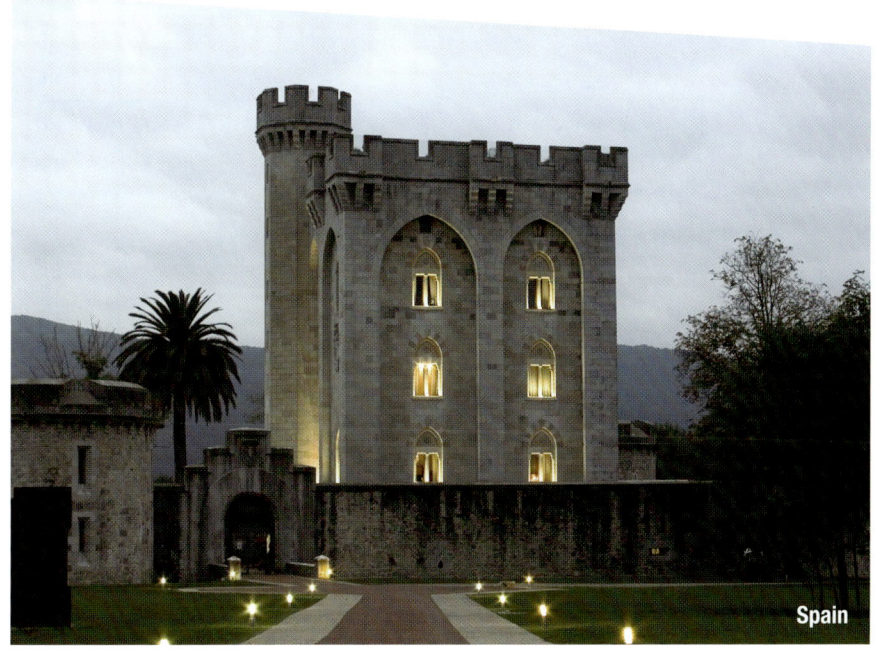

Chile

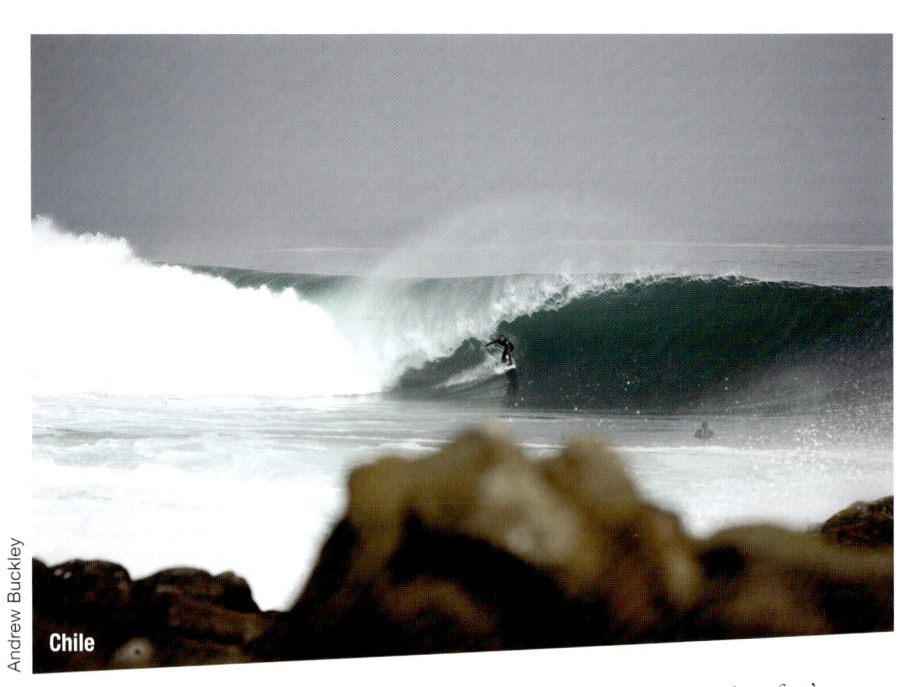

The cold slab of El Gringo's in the northern Chile desert tested surfers' skills like never before in WCT competition. Above, Kieren Perrow eyes the escape. Below, an empty wave breaks on the shallow ledge. If this is too much, you can easily escape down south for the famous point breaks in greener pastures.

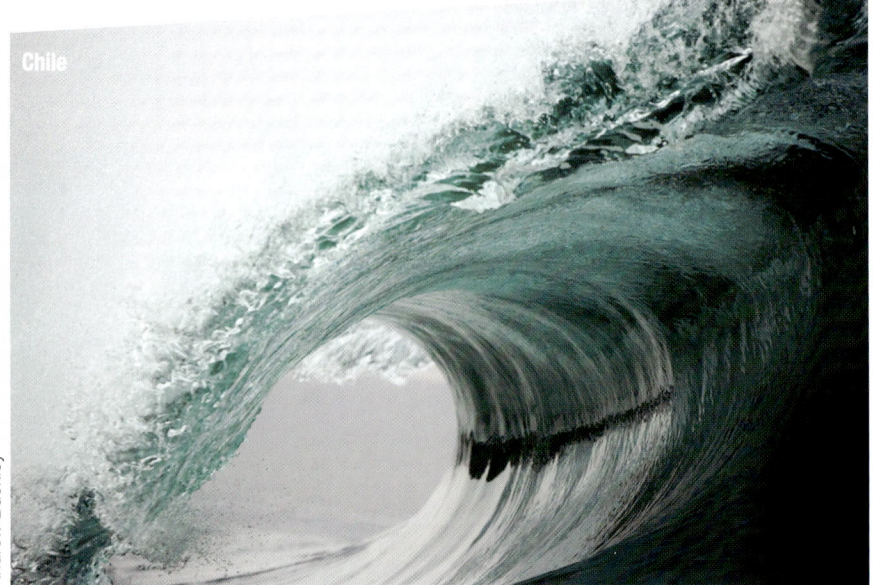

Chile

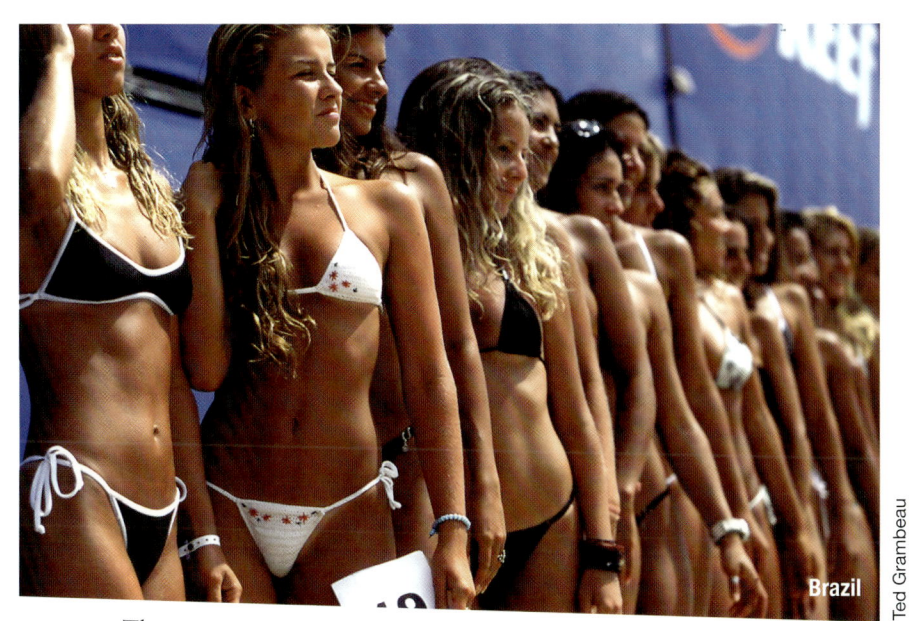

The attraction of Brazil isn't always the waves.

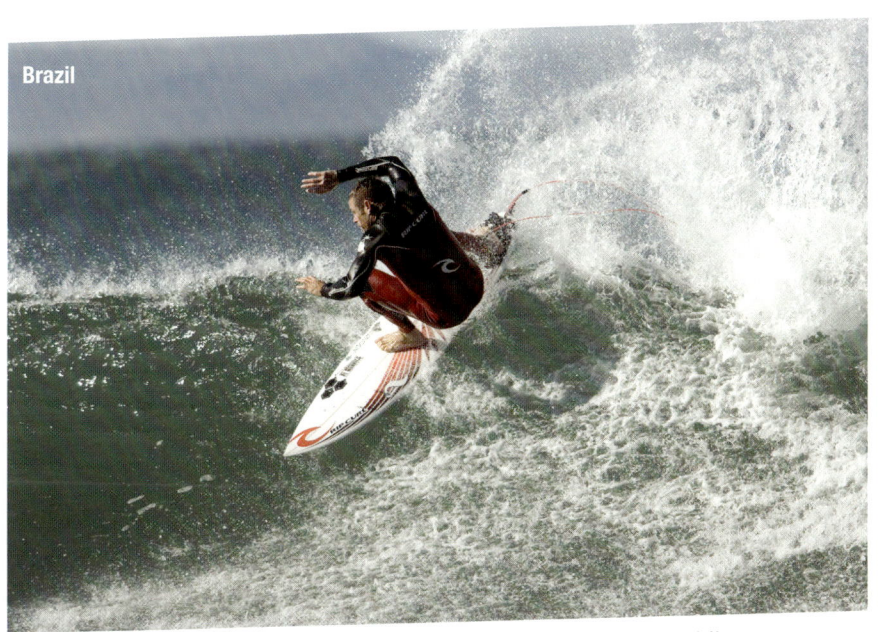

Taylor Knox: technician, powerhouse and one of the world's most-respected surfers.

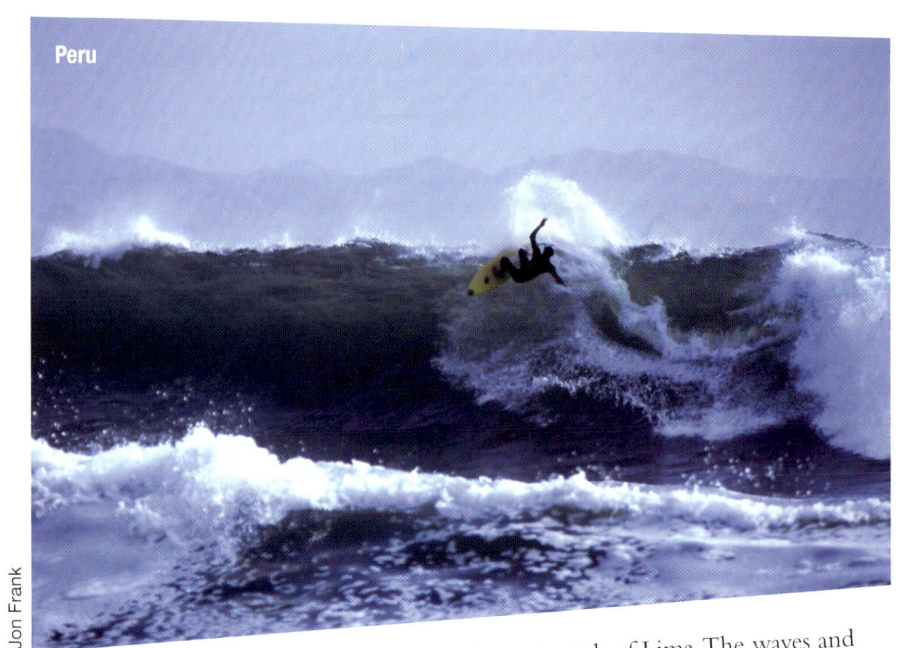

Rasta cuts through a right-hand point south of Lima. The waves and culture have travelled a long way to get to this mysterious place.

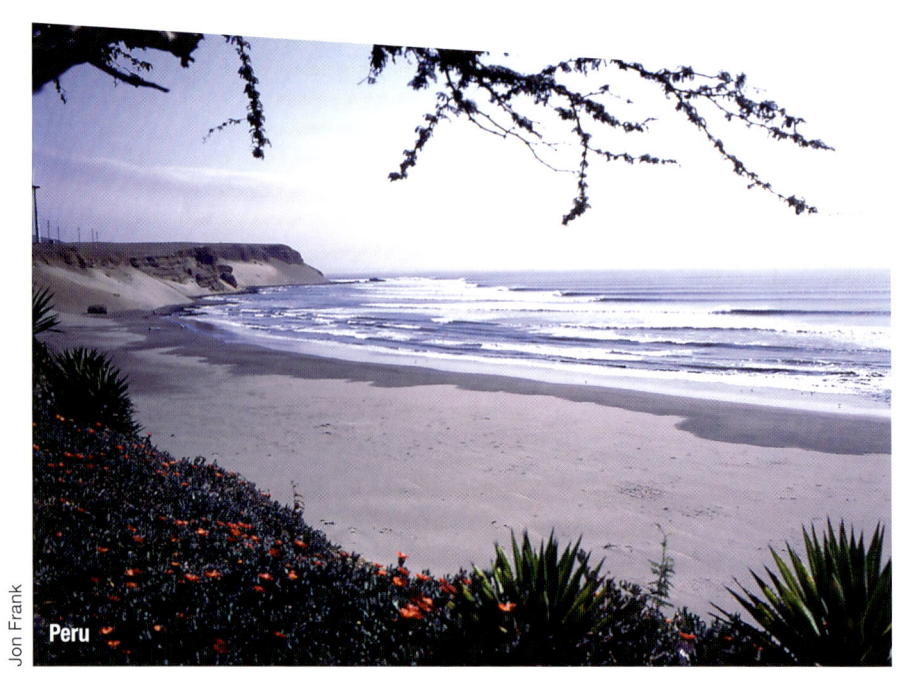

The famous lineup of Chicama … the world's longest left.

observe that the place seems to be just falling over itself to be more like America, and not in a good way.

'England differs from the rest of the world in that nowhere else has made such a contribution to the global soundscape. Possibly due to the ugly weather, for decades Brits have gone indoors and made music whose global reach has been unprecedented. Look at the size of the country on a globe and then consider the influence in terms of bands, artists and genres. Nowhere else even comes close. Because of this, football and the language have always given us a higher global profile than most similarly sized nations.'

We surfed a lot on our trips to England, mostly around Newquay. Anyone studying surfing at the University of Plymouth would tell you that the obtuse gradient of the coast spilling into the ocean slows the swells before they become waves. They are so slow that it's almost as if they have had to come uphill. They tend to roll from far away and re-form with the power of the wind swells. There are some surfing events in England and some great surfers — like Russell Winter, who made the WCT — but for most it still remains a dream encapsulated in surf mags. However, the dream is easily accessible due to the proximity of one of the world's busiest airports and one of the world's strongest currencies. In the meantime, surfing in England merely keeps the salt on your skin, the timing on your board and the feeling at an accessible point until the next sojourn.

'The standard of surfing I guess is okay relative to the conditions,' said Paul. 'There are good surfers all over but few great surfers. For the vast majority of people, surfing in England will remain an experience sport rather than a performance one. What I'd like to see is surfing as a positive lifestyle choice, rather than any surges for ASP greatness. If more Brits develop a love of surfing and the coast, not only will it be good for the health and wellbeing of individuals and society, but also for the coastal environment itself.'

In the summer, between gaps in the grey, the Brits swarm the beach. There are festivals boasting the nation's top artists in every genre. It all goes on despite the grey; they dance and laugh beneath it. In these moments you get a glimpse of the Great in Great Britain — and of the wealth they have exported to civilised nations all around the world. From small islands off Antarctica to the biggest island in the world, from David Beckham, the Beatles and the Rolling Stones to Shakespeare — its name is associated with them all. Great Britain's influence is unmatched. However, if there is one more thing they would wish to export, it would be the omnipresent grey that blankets them, the bedspread that has made them who they are.

I was in a pub in Plymouth. The beer was a little warmer than I'm used to and the jokes a little funnier. Outside, waves whipped across the harbour and a small child struggled to keep the pastie in his hands. Seagulls complained at his selfishness. The geezers inside had given up peering out the window for the day and the sun was about to give up trying to push through as well. Inside, the patrons were singing and laughing, telling jokes, throwing darts and playing pool. They talked of the royal family like it was part of their own bloodline; they embraced their history and reflected on their achievements with pride. A weather report came on the TV, watched eagerly by the patrons. But if the sun can't make its way through the grey on the morrow — and it probably won't, despite it being the middle of summer — if it can't spill colour on the Mother Country, they will find their own colour. They will stare down their only worthy foe and sing with pride and laughter, 'Look at the scoreboard.'

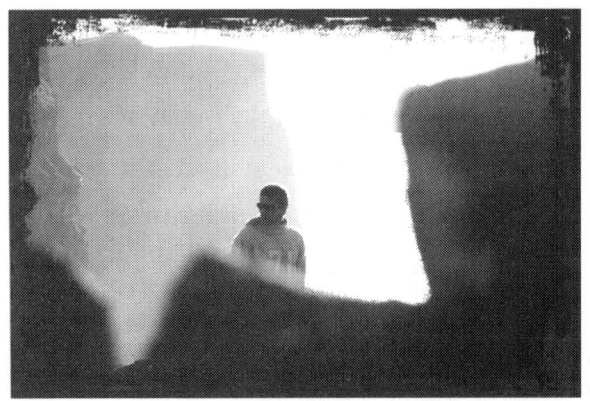

## ... AND THEN THE WIND STOPPED
### IRELAND

It was in the rolling green hills of Ireland that I starting looking for the four-leaf clover. As fate would have it, I found a few other things along the way I also considered lucky: powerful reef breaks, tepid beers and a warm-natured jovial people. In some strange way, all of this consolidated an already existing feeling of connection to Ireland. I don't consider this to be unique to me. Why is it that wherever you go in this world, there's some connection with Ireland? Maybe it's her raw landscape we connect with. Maybe it's the powerful ocean that speaks to the wild side of our nature. Maybe it's the country's history, the struggle with authority — because we always like the underdog. Or, more likely, it's a family tree. If you're from America, New Zealand or Australia, chances are that the roots of your family tree are planted in a village in Ireland. Even if you don't have roots in the four-leaf clover, Ireland evokes a feeling that leaves you wishing you did.

## WHAT THE MAN IN THE PUB RECKONS

He wasn't a celebrated historian, but he'd told a few stories over the years. And what he lost in facts, he made up for with clever delivery and timely jokes. Castles, swords, Vikings, warm coats and funny accents ... It was in a pub in Dublin that I first engaged in warm beer and conversation with Michael, a construction worker, who, like the majority of his fellow countrymen, was enjoying a beer that Friday afternoon.

'Celtic tribes arrived on the island between 600–150 BC,' said Michael between sips of Guinness. 'Must have been bloody cold!' He looked around the bar and up to the television which was showing a game of Gaelic football between Meath and Westmeath. It was a huge clash. 'The English started invading in the twelfth century and ...' He rubbed his fists together like two mismatched pieces of a jigsaw puzzle. 'We have an interesting history. There were rebellions. One failed in 1916 — the Easter Monday Rebellion, it was.' His eyes wandered north, searching both the left and right sides of his brain for information and clever stories to fill the gap. 'Then there was more fighting, several years of guerrilla warfare that gave us independence from the United Kingdom in 1921. But it was only for twenty-six southern counties. You see, Ireland is made up of thirty-two counties. The six northern [Ulster] counties remained part of the United Kingdom. So that is what the fuss is all about — the IRA, the bombs and the songs from U2.'

In 1948 Ireland withdrew from the British Commonwealth and in 1973 joined the European Community. Irish governments have sought the peaceful unification of Ireland and have cooperated with Britain against terrorist groups. A peace settlement for Northern Ireland is being implemented with great difficulty. The situation has provoked years of passion and pride, and inspired many books and movies about mankind's ongoing battle with authority, the need for independence, and the desire to evolve uninhibited. It doesn't matter whether you're a person or a country — you want to run your own show, right?

## ... AND THEN THE WIND STOPPED

A solitary surfer walking along an Irish beach, board in hand, looking for waves is not an uncommon sight these days. But on a cold spring day in 1963, it was a sight that locals had never seen before. Ian Hill — possibly Ireland's first surfer — had found his four-leaf clover when he had seen surfing in Cornwall, England and knew it was for him. He bought a board from an Australian lifeguard and, with that purchase, imported surfing to Ireland. While he now carries the booty of four decades of surfing knowledge, it didn't start that way. He had no wetsuits; he didn't even know you had to put wax on the board.

'We couldn't get wetsuits. I can remember getting a sheet of neoprene, lying on top of it and having my aunt draw around me to get the shape before gluing it together. It was primitive by today's standards, but an improvement on jeans and a T-shirt.'

By the mid-seventies, there were around twenty surfers in Ireland, among them Alan Duke, the first Irish champion. While there are a lot more surfers now, it's still pretty easy to get a wave to yourself, especially on the challenging reef breaks, as most locals can't surf at that level yet. While they have the wetsuit technology now, the water is still freezing; winds can lash the coast for weeks on end and the plethora of shallow ledges make the entry level appealing only to extremists. But every now and again the wind stops, leaving opportunities to find a different kind of clover. One surfer who saw this potential was American big wave charger Rusty Long. His pioneering of the Lahinch coast awoke a sleeping beast.

## AILL NA SEARRACH

It is one of Ireland's greatest and most popular tourist attractions: the Cliffs of Moher on the west coast of Ireland. Of an almost incomprehensible size, the cliffs are massive and menacing, dropping vertically from the clouds into the ocean. It's nature at its most intense and your first peer over the edge stirs the stomach. It seems like the edge of the world and I'm sure that ancient cultures shared this opinion. For years the number of tourists multiplied, all eager for the towering spectacle, the raw tenacity, that is the Cliffs of Moher.

Sometime in its history, a section of rock fell from the cliff, creating a break for massive waves. Surfers are an unusual breed in Ireland, but it would take an even rarer type to notice the wave down there and then entertain the idea of surfing it. But in 2004, some bodyboarders made the first Everest-like attempt.

'Can you believe it?' asked Gavin Gallagher, who's making a film about surfing in Ireland. 'This wave was there the whole time — and nobody even noticed it. Then when they did, the problem was how to actually get down there. Because the cliffs are so high and vertical, there's no way to get down.' Imagine a rock wall around 200 metres high and you have the Cliffs of Moher. It was a conundrum for even the most cunning of surfers, but soon enough somebody found a way.

'The first guys to surf it were a couple of bodyboarders,' said Gavin. He paused to add dramatic effect to the following sentence. 'They paddled three and a half kilometres to the break from the closest entry point in a nearby town.' He paused again, excited by a story he had obviously rehearsed. 'By the time they got there — about six hours later — it was dark and they had to turn back. But because there was no town, no lights and the stars were behind the clouds, it was pitch black and they were as good as lost at sea. Luckily, they had a mate on top of the cliffs with a cigarette lighter.' Their mate kept the small cigarette lighter burning, lighting the way back to safety, while the bodyboarders kicked and paddled through the dark and dangerous water. Their waveless journey finished six kilometres and ten hours after it started.

Then on 15 October 2005 Rusty Long became the first person to surf the wave, partnering up with local surfers John McCarthy (the current Irish champion) and Dave Blount. 'I'd known about the wave and had been watching it for a little while,' said Rusty, who spends the better part of most days on his computer tracking massive swells. 'I was trying to work out the ideal conditions. I saw a massive swell building in the Atlantic, the winds looked favourable, so I bombed it over there.' The wind had stopped! Rusty scored some epic waves and opened another chapter in big wave surfing.

'It is a very impressive wave. It sucks out of really deep water and peaks up on this ledge. For sure it's going to be one of the most hardcore big wave spots in the world today. I've been watching it ever since, because I think it can hold a lot bigger. I think it can hold anything!'

I ventured down the cliff one sunny afternoon, and while the swell was only around six foot and nowhere near big enough to break, it seemed like the land of the giants. Nothing will ever happen in small portions here, and as more surfers like Rusty come to the cliffs, you'll hear more and more about this sleeping giant.

The wave's name is Aill Na Searrach and the legend around it tells a story of how white horses ran and threw themselves over the cliffs. Today, the white horses remain in the form of howling white caps galloping on the wind back to shore, and when the wind stops, there will be more surfers throwing themselves over the cliffs in their own semi-suicidal pursuit.

## THE WEEPING WIDOW

The rock of the family unit, embodied in a statue, celebrates the enduring story of the fisherman's wife. Her symbol stands tall against the westerly coast, as the wind and rain attempt to blow her down. She stands defiant against the elements. Her cement dress is fixed in a flow behind her, as if frozen on the coldest and windiest of winter days. For months her husband goes to sea in the wild ocean to catch his fish and earn his bread, and her arms are outstretched, waiting for him to return. 'The Weeping Widow' is the historic talisman of an enduring pain — the hope that her husband will come home safe from the sea. But it didn't always work out that way. As an alarming percentage of fishermen are lost at sea, the hoping widow became the weeping widow. Bodies would consistently wash up onto the hard western shore, unrecognisable even to the wives. So the women started knitting individual patterns on their husbands' jumpers, so that in the event that their husbands washed ashore, they would recognise the pattern on their knitwear — and therefore their husbands. She waits … and hopes … but all too often she weeps.

## FOREIGN INVESTMENT

The two Tylers came from different parts of the globe for the same reasons — adventure and experience. Surfing and good times made up the other two leaves in their clover. One from Australia and the other from California, they never knew each other previously, but they now shared an apartment in Lahinch, working, surfing and living the Irish dream. I met them on my first surf in Ireland. They surfed well and knew the area.

'It's fun here,' said the Australian Tyler. 'There's something pretty cool about running over a green hill, past cows and an ancient castle for a surf. There are always parties! Fuck, man, they drink so much here! There's an excuse every day to drink, but the people are so much fun you can't help but jump on the bandwagon. It's a good place to work and save money too. I'm a builder and I've done a bit of work in construction, but I don't have all my tools with me and for most jobs you need to have your own tools. So I started to coach people how to surf in the local surf school in Lahinch. It's growing so much. There are always customers and people who want to learn, even when it's cold and windy. The wages are good and because you're paid in pounds, you can travel on that currency and take some money home.'

They both plan on staying for at least a year. 'Yeah, I'm going to see out the winter,' said the American Tyler. 'This place is unreal. The waves are great, the people are so friendly. I ain't going anywhere in a hurry.'

## THE PUB

In Lahinch there's a man who owns a good old Irish pub. Rumour has it, he pours a better Guinness than anyone. And so he should — he's been doing it for eighty-two years! He is eighty-nine years old and has been working behind the bar since he was a kid. 'I first started pouring beers when I was seven — and have ever since. I only have two days off a year — Christmas and Good Friday — and I am the only one who works here, ever.' He was proud of his work ethic. 'The bar hasn't changed one bit since I started.' Looking around, I saw tins of custard that could be older than him sitting behind the bar. The wooden shelves, like him, have cracked and wrinkled with age, and they leaned on each other for support. His frail body, just like his bar, held a hint of corrosion, but they seemed to hold each other up pretty well. It was an old relationship and they understood each other. As he walked around, his body cracked like the hard wood floor beneath his step. If you peered behind the fogged and scratched lens of the right side of his reading glasses, you would see that he was missing an eye. I wasn't even sure if the other one worked.

I watched him try and plug in his wireless. It took him minutes to find the power point, which was only an arms-length away. I soon realised then that he was blind, but he was so used to his own bar, he didn't miss a beat and probably didn't even need his sight. He ran his fingers along the bar as if reading braille and felt his way to the tap — the Guinness tap; the only one there. He poured us a beer. It was the best Guinness in Ireland, poured purely by feel — a feel that resides within all Irish.

### DAMO

It was an average summer day in Ireland; the rising sun cast an orange glow that teased the early morning frost with false hopes of warmth. The wind held the promise of breaking the glorious view in front of me with the omnipresent delivery of clouds. The sky was mostly blue, but that could change very quickly. It was time to move. Rusty Long had told me about some quality ledges in the Lahinch area, so I put two steamers, a pair of booties, a towel, a raincoat and my hopes in the back of my car and headed out. My first day of surfing here and getting back into a wet wetsuit had taught me to be better prepared for day two. I joined up with Gavin Gallagher and one of the new generation of sponsored surfers coming through the Irish ranks, Damien (Damo) Conway.

At sixteen years old, Damo is your typical grommet; long blond hair, confident, cheeky, brash. He is also one of the first real hopes that Ireland has of competing internationally.

Damo had taken off early from school so he could surf with us. We drove down the coast road past reef ledges and exposed beaches and picked him up from his school. He was excited to be going surfing with us and we chatted in the car about his four-leaf clover.

'My sister had a board and I borrowed it and learned that way. Then I got my own. The waves here are great, but sometimes it can be flat all summer. And then when the waves do come, it's usually windy, so it can be frustrating because the weather decides when you can surf around here.'

Although young, he had a certain maturity and wisdom, and I found myself listening intently.

'You can be so keen to surf sometimes. Like I'll watch a surf movie and get really excited to surf, but you can't even walk outside the house or you'll get blown away!

'It's so cold too: 5/4s are a minimum in winter and you need booties and a hood as well. You can wear 3/2 in summer, but you still have your cold days.'

We surfed an outer bomby, and Damo surfed quite well. But he knows he'll need to travel to get to the next level. 'We have domestic competitions, but I go to England and sometimes to France to go in Pro Juniors. I want to surf as much as I can and keep getting better. It's a hard thing to do here. The level is pretty high, but we just don't get to surf enough because of the weather. But every now and again — the wind stops.'

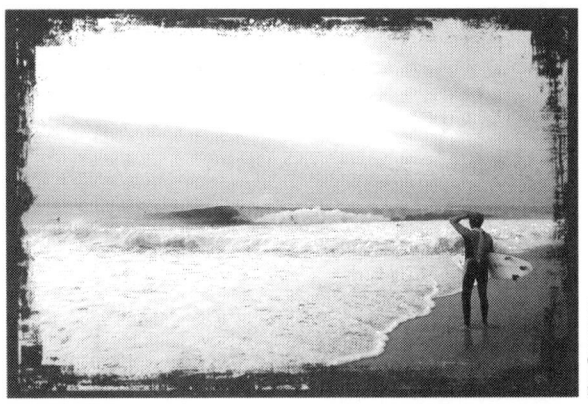

# VIVE LE OUI
## FRANCE

Visiting France can be quite inspiring if you take into account three things. First, they have a culture of intense respect for intellectuals. Second, their ladies are world champion lovers; they are incredibly beautiful, displaying a femininity as if descended from Venus herself. They also have a comfortable affinity with nudity, which is very alluring. Third, next to the rolling green hills at the foot of the Pyrenees Mountains and the French Alps, there is an ocean of pumping waves. People have been invading France for years — and you can't blame them. From armies to tourists, people from all around the world have come to France. Still, it remains one of the strongest cultures on the planet, impenetrable to dilution and a romantic inspiration to everyone. But before I go too far, one aspect of their culture needs to be explained.

## ARROGANCE?

It is widely accepted that the French possess a reputation for arrogance — a strong feeling of proud self-importance that is expressed by treating other people with contempt or disregard. Simply translated: they truly believe the way they conduct their lives, the way they speak, cook, eat and root is vastly superior to that of other nations. Let's dive into this straight away, so you don't read this story through fixed glasses.

Without growing a moustache and waving a French flag, I'd have to admit that their food is superior; their language more precise in its poetry; their daily life, which doesn't bend to capitalism like most Western countries, remarkable; and that they don't root — they make love. Holidays are holidays — and at lunch you sleep. No matter how many wallets are knocking on your business door, siesta time is siesta time. Arrogance? It depends on your interpretation. They have one of the highest life expectancy rates in the world and a rich culture. The fact that their country is visited by more tourists than any other indicates that perhaps we all appreciate this. Why else would we go there?

Aurelie Laborde was my girlfriend for a year or two. She had beautiful big eyes, soft feminine features, a full set of curves and an accent that could melt the wax off my board. She was also as French as they come and my real introduction to French culture.

Sleeping till lunchtime was normal. Orange juice, coffee and baguette for breakfast (traditional French breakfast): normal. She'll lie on the beach on her days off work, drink coffee and siesta when the weather doesn't permit outside excursions, pottering around without expending too much energy. One time she had to set her alarm for lunch with her dad at 12 pm.

She smoked cigarettes because it was 'her pleasure' and indulged in meals like marathons that consisted of aperitifs, entrees, digestives and desserts every day.

'Everybody [in France] learns languages for seven years at school,' she said. 'It's not that they are rude or arrogant, I don't think; maybe sometimes, but we are shy to speak it in case we get it wrong. We are lazy at everything except the language.'

I once told her I had a bad crème brulee in Tahiti. She said, 'Just because they can speak French doesn't mean they can cook it.'

Correct pronunciation, manners and taste were a prerequisite for the way Aurelie lived her life. She was funny, she was feminine, she was … French.

## FULL BELLY

Belly was one of the first Australian surfers to go to France. Originally known as Stephen Bell, 'Belly' grew up in Torquay, Victoria. He was invited by a mate to go and check out the southwest of France and he has lived there ever since: twenty-two years. He even speaks the language now.

'I'd want to be able to speak the language,' he laughed. 'If I didn't when I first got here, I wouldn't be able to talk. It was either learn French, or don't talk.' For Belly, it was a new start; he'd just lost his father and needed some direction.

'There was nobody here back then in 1985. It was just a tiny little holiday village and nobody knew anything about surfing, because nobody surfed.' Belly lives in a little villa house on the beach in Hossegor — and the barbecue is always fired, the coffee fresh and the beer fridge always open for every travelling Aussie surfer. His Aussie accent is also intact.

Belly works for Quiksilver now, managing the affairs of Kelly Slater and others on tour. I get to spend a lot of time with him, since we have similar jobs (if you can call them that). On that day, as we chatted about his life in France, we were playing golf on Hossegor — one of the oldest golf courses in the country. The houses at the edges of the course were hundreds of years old, seemingly carved out of the forest. They had both been there for so long that they were now a part of each other. The smell of pine trees and the hint of salt in the sea breeze suggested the ocean was close by.

The village hasn't changed much since Belly moved there. A little coastal village with a small population that swells with tourists in summer, it has been going about its business for hundreds of years. And with regards to the French surfing scene, the only thing that existed when Belly first arrived were the waves. It was a good place to start.

'I originally came out to start making surfboards here as the market was developing and nobody really knew how; everything was imported.' Thus Euroglass was born — Belly's business — and his contribution to the development of surfing in France and Europe.

'I surfed by myself for a long time. I always used to wonder where all those boards I made went to. We'd make so many, yet you'd never see anyone in the surf. Now I see them all. There are so many more surfers now. It's exploded! We can't keep up.'

Surfboards are now walking out the door quicker than baguettes from a bakery. And as Paris is the capital for fashion and all things romantic, Hossegor in the south is the belly button of all things surfing. The industry is there, the surfers are there. This is due to the generally universal reason — the omnipresent magnet for all surfers — waves.

The Bay of Biscay is built for surf. Low-pressure systems form in the North Atlantic below Greenland and follow the conveyor belt that is the North Atlantic current towards Europe. The bay itself is very deep, and doesn't rise until the swells crash suddenly on shallow sandbanks right on the shoreline. It means the waves don't slow down and you get Hawaii-like power. It's home to the Quiksilver Pro, one of the most anticipated stops on the ASP World Tour. Anyone from Europe who wants to surf and experience the ocean generally comes to the south of France.

All this happens on the 200-kilometre stretch of coast between Biarritz and Bordeaux, an area better known for wine. There are no bays, points, coves or inlets; just one very, very long beach with mountains of sand dunes to disperse the banks as the currents see fit. So if you can find an access point through the forest, you can discover uncrowded waves at any spot. The area from Biarritz to Bordeaux is actually one giant sand dune. In fact, it used to be swamp and marshland, until one of the Napoleons planted thousands of pine trees, which created the forest that is there today.

Belly pointed to the trees all around the golf course. 'These thirsty trees drink up to 250 litres of water a day. It was a pretty good idea, because this land was uninhabitable before.' Soon the land was stabilised and ready for habitation. Napoleon built his wife a castle on the beach in Biarritz — and the endless supply of sand provided the endless supply of surf. So was born the south of France.

## LOVING LAZY

Biarritz is a place that has it all. It is at the foot of the Pyrenees, and freshwater rivers flow between the green mountains and hills that line the sandy shores. The salt air finds its way through the ancient streets past cafes and restaurants. The historic castles and houses lend character to the chic cosmopolitan way of life. It is truly one of the most attractive places in the world. The waves pump, the city life is exciting — and all around, the beauty of nature is overwhelming.

'There are only 250,000 people in Biarritz,' said Robert, a local from the area. 'That is not too many people — and not many of these people surf. When we first started to surf, it was considered a weird thing to do. There was society — and then there were surfers. Now it is a huge sport involving lots of money so the local people are into it now.'

Robert has seen it all. He has also travelled the world, so he can draw careful comparisons. If you've ever been to France, or spoken to someone who has, you'll know that the surfers are different there.

'In France we are very lazy. The people look at the waves and if it's not offshore, they are not going out.' He laughs. 'It's the same if there is a rip or the waves are closing out — we are not going out. In Australia I notice that everybody gets up really early to surf. I see on the Gold Coast that there are fifty people out when the sun comes up. You are not going to see this in France. We are sleeping.

'In Spain, for example, they wear a helmet and charge the big waves on the reef breaks. They have the hot blood. They fight the bulls — and that is how they surf.' He laughs again. 'Not the French. If the waves are too big, we are not going out. Of course, this doesn't apply to everybody. Some people look for big waves and like to surf by themselves, but for the most part, French surfers are like — how you say — sheep?'

'They're world champion checkers, mate,' said Richard 'Dog' Marsh. Dog grew up in Cronulla in Sydney, where he lived with his French wife,

Sabine, for over fifteen years before she convinced the family to move back to her homeland.

'I just wanted our kids to learn French while they were still young, and experience the culture,' she said.

'I go out early and there's nobody around,' said Dog. Then you come in and there are ten or twenty people checking it. Maybe it's too cold, or there are a couple of closeouts. They don't go out. And it's pumping, mate, proper eight-foot barrels, and they go, "Oh, there are some closeouts; maybe I go later." It's so funny.'

Dog is good friends with Robert, who he met through Sabine as they both grew up in Anglet. I stay back there after Mundaka finishes every year and it's my favourite time of year. Everyone has gone home — the surfers, the tourists — and you get to see who the locals are, what sort of place it is and experience the culture undiluted by foreign influence. What's more, the waves are pumping and everybody is ... checking it.

## LA FEMININE

'It is because we are more chic.' Her answer to my question was pretty funny. I figured that getting a couple of girls together to talk about all things feminine in France might give an insight into their way of life — and their way of putting life in both the hearts and trousers of men.

Cloe, Aurelie and Claire grew up in Hossegor; they watch their town turn into a tourist monster every summer and endure its sleepy, cold winters. They like the excitement of the summer — the international flavour — and they usually chase it in the winter, flying around the world to somewhere 'exotic'. They are all hot — but 'hot' or 'sexy' are not words they like — or a description they aspire to — in France. 'We don't want to be sexy like a slut,' said

Aurelie. 'I hate that! We try to be beautiful. It is much better for a girl. Much more chic!'

'When I was growing up I didn't know about the rest of the world,' said Claire. 'I thought France was everything, but then all the people started coming. It's just a small town, but it gets so busy. All the French and Parisians come in August, then people from all around the world. Then everyone goes. I love the place and I love the people coming because it makes it more exciting. But when everyone goes, it is like a ghost town and we get so bored. We just sleep.'

The girls grew up working in the hospitality industry, serving *moules* (mussels) at Capreton. After work they go out, sleep in late, go back to work and start it all over again. That's how they live during the summer. 'I just want to lay on the beach, sleep, have a good dinner, then have a party. That is perfect.' But when things die down and the international visitors leave, they get more opportunities to experience their own country.

'My cousin grew up in the French Basque country,' said Claire. 'She doesn't even speak French — only Basque. Her family lives off the farm and I went there this year. It was so weird! We killed a pig. You shoot this metal stick through its brain, and then you have meat for one year. They make the sausage, *jambon* [ham] — everything. Then we killed a duck. You boil it and make something from every part; some part for pâté, some for foie gras. It was so cool.'

The girls have tried surfing, but much prefer to just lie on the beach.

'We are very different. It is not like in Australia or America where all the girls exercise and have the big boobs. We are lazy. We sleep in, never exercise. But I think we dress more feminine. It is all in the details,' she laughed. 'It is our culture to have long meals and just talk. For sure we are different.'

'*Oui*, we are more chic,' repeated Aurelie. I remember one night in Australia when I was teasing Aurelie, saying, 'I'll leave you here and you can walk home.' She just replied with confidence, 'I can just go to any man and say, "Excuse me, but I am French and I am lost. Can you please help me?"' Somewhere behind that beautiful accent, the feminine dress and the chic attitude, French girls can have anyone by the balls.

## A YARN

Not all locals are sheep — and not all come from the famous area between Biarritz and Hossegor in the French Basque country. Yann Martin is from Lacanau — another little coastal village that flares in the summer — at the end of the sand dune and just off the coast of Bordeaux. In Lacanau you can find everything from some of the earliest traces of human existence to the finest of French wines. It was there that the makers of Champagne got together to ban the use of that word by anyone else around the world. Arrogance? Again, it depends on your interpretation, but from now on, unless it is made in France, Champagne is called 'sparkling white wine'. It is also where a lot of holidaymakers and surfers make their way.

'One time I was in the water in Lacanau with some tourists, and one of the guys was on all the waves,' said Yann. 'I just told him that it was a friendly spot and when we give him some waves he must wait his turn. This guy told me, "Hey man, I'm a local here so go home." At that time I had a house right on the beach. I just pointed to my house and told him, "Good start, bru."'

There are a lot of foreigners now living in France, including many Australians and English. They add to the melting pot of cultures and colours. But at the end of the day, the French culture is way too strong to be diluted — and it can be hard to fit in. 'The locals are starting to get pissed off,' Aurelie told me once. 'Because all the Australians are coming to France and taking the waves, the jobs and all the girls.'

All of this has always happened in summer, which they are used to. But now people are staying on after the season. When the sleepy little coastal towns of Hossegor and Lacanau draw their shutters, close their shops and the commercial world hibernates, the tourists aren't going. This is generally when the waves get better too.

Yann has seen it all. He is one of the original surfers of Lacanau — and all of France — and a former three-time French champ. Over the years he has seen the local surfing culture grow into the massive machine it is today. After his stint in the army in 1989, he began to surf in Lacanau, competing and collecting almost every trophy you could in France, before the foreigners started coming.

'Surfing was different back then, because nobody did it, so it was very friendly. Now the culture, the industry — everything has changed. Well, not the culture. The culture is still the same, because it's just about riding waves and being in the ocean. But the industry is completely different. Today, surfing is more of a business and it is much more professional. A lot of guys who work in the surf industry are not surfers and the image has changed here in Europe.'

With the extra professionalism has come extra talent. Guys like Micky Picon led the way for a while. He was talented, and qualified for the World Championship Tour in 2006, but he never really took it all the way.

'There is also a lot of money here now and I think we pay our surfers too much — it makes them lazy,' said Yann.

It's true; these guys can get paid healthy sums to stay at home, dominate the European Tour, surf great waves and never leave Europe. It looks as though Jeremy Flores will be the first one to change that. He won the WQS in 2006 and, in his first year on tour, finished in the top ten, becoming rookie of the year. He's a good surfer. He goes hard, isn't scared of losing or winning, and isn't lazy — therefore he's hard to beat. There are more surfers beneath him, rising through the ranks.

Surfing is in its infancy, but it is at the dawn of a growth spurt. It may not be strong enough to get most of the French up for the early, or to paddle through closeouts, but it is running through France like a blitzkrieg, through the cafes and small villages and onto the sandy beaches where nude bathers don't just come to the south of France to bask, they come to surf. In their own way, the French culture of artisans is making love with the new culture of surfing.

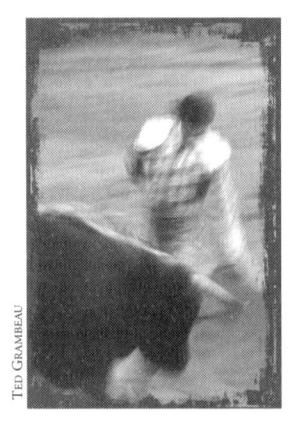

# FROM ETA TO EUCALYPT
## SPAIN

Borders are odd things; they mark territory, keep people out, keep people in, define people, their language, their culture and their government. Sometimes borders are decided by war, sometimes by diplomacy. They are an indication of man's preoccupation with measuring things and ownership. However, sometimes geography itself is strong enough to make that decision.

When you drive over the border from southern France to the north of Spain, the changes are abrupt. One minute you're saying '*Merci beaucoup*', for the change from the tollbooth to a cute-looking French lady; five minutes down the road, the building is a different colour, the people have dark hair, usually in a mullet, and they deliver their thanks swiftly with a lisping '*Gracias*'.

You have entered a new world of geographic, linguistic and cultural contrast. The geography has suddenly become mountainous — you are at the feet of the Pyrenees — and towns congregate around a church square. There's an extra fire in the people's blood — a passion for something that is way older than the borders that imprison them. I say that because the population here believe in borders that existed long before their current confines, borders of a place that once extended into France and the hills of the Pyrenees. As soon as you cross the border, everyone is talking about the 'Basque country'.

## PROTECTING THE PAST

They say here that 'Before God was God and boulders were boulders, Basques were already Basques'. The language is over 500 years old, and, like their society and their culture, is from a time before the arrival of even the Indo-Europeans to this area. Their culture has survived and endured many wars and many rulers; it has hidden in the hills like a seed, always regenerating. The Basque people are fierce about protecting their past, one of the most beautiful and traditional of all Europe. You don't have to go to a museum to see it; it is evident in everyday life and plain to see, but not, however, recognised by governments or borders.

Out of this culture a movement was born — Euskadi Ta Askatasuna or ETA (Basque for 'Basque Homeland and Freedom' — an armed Basque nationalist separatist organisation. Founded in 1959, it has evolved from asking for cultural recognition to demanding it. To date, since 1968, the ETA has killed 821 people and committed dozens of kidnappings. More than 500 ETA members are incarcerated in prisons in Spain, France and other countries. Some of them are surfers. ETA is described as a terrorist organisation by both the Spanish and French authorities as well as by the European Union as a whole, the United States and the United Nations. With such a reputation, you'd imagine the movement would be underground, beneath the social setting. But it's not. All over the towns of Basque Spain, like Burneo, San Sebastian, and even Bilbao, there are footprints of the ETA. There are rallies, graffiti on walls, and explosions in government buildings.

That's the harsh side. Then there is the beautiful side — kids and their parents wearing the green and red berets, talking in their traditional language and participating in cultural activities like *pilota*.

'The Basque country has been around for a long time,' said Aneko Acero, Basque professional surfer. 'It's such an old culture and has been around way before Spain was. A lot of the people want to keep this culture and to have it recognised.'

At the centre of the Basque country is a small coastal fishing village. It wears the green and red in its shop windows, in the tapas bars and on the masts of boats that, every morning, sail past what could be the best left in the world.

## MUNDAKA

When the west coast of Europe suddenly turns into a north coast, like an L turned back to front, you are in the Basque country of Spain. You might have heard of San Sebastian, renowned for its hundreds of tapas bars and historical setting. Just a little further west is Mundaka. The drive there was pleasant on the eyes, but hard on the equilibrium, as we rounded the series of hairpin corners over rugged mountains and green hilltops. All the while, the view from the cliff top revealed old churches on rocky islands and waves crashing against their rugged walls.

'I have been surfing here for twenty-eight years,' said one of the older generation from Bakio, a small beach with a bigger town just twenty minutes away from Mundaka. He won the first event here in '87, and was one of the first to surf this famous wave. 'Back then, we used to park our cars right on the point and all of this —' His hands made dismissive gestures towards the surrounding park and boardwalk, the human veneer that sits over this natural amphitheatre. All around were cafes, courtyards and the *pilota* court where the men play in traditional dress. 'Back then, I couldn't find anyone to surf with, but now if it's good, there are hundreds of people out.'

What a true statement. Only one year earlier when we had been here, the surf was pumping, almost as good as it gets, and all the surfers of the Quiksilver Pro in France, which had been called off due to massive waves, had made the journey to surf Mundaka. Hossegor was at least twelve to fifteen foot and this translates to six foot plus at Mundaka. The big valley that borders the river steers the wind offshore to its mouth, holding up some of the longest and most perfect barrels I've ever seen.

'Mundaka has to be the best wave on the planet,' Tom Curren said as we paddled out, watching Kelly Slater get a fifteen-second barrel. When we viewed some of the footage later, it wasn't even the longest tube. Nathan Hedge had clocked in one at seventeen seconds, more or less from start to finish. The banks were good that day, but it's not always that way.

'Since the dredging last year, the sand has moved,' said Zugui Zegarra, a local surfing champ. 'For a while, the waves weren't even breaking here. They did the dredging because there was so much sand that the boats couldn't make it through the river. But they took so much sand that even the biggest swells weren't breaking.'

A year since that last visit, we sat wondering if Mother Nature was going to produce the goods for the Billabong Pro. The sand was even starting to come back, despite fears that it was lost forever.

Zugui looked over the break towards the dramatic sea cliffs in the background. The sand was back, but the waves here are fickle; even when they do come, you can only surf them through low tide.

'This is a hot day, too hot for October,' he said. 'The onshore will be here in less than an hour, I'd bet my house on it!' The wind hit before we could finish our coffee. The event was called off for the day and we surfed at Bakio.

Zugui makes surfboards for a living. Well, he used to make surfboards, but times have changed since the early eighties when he first started surfing here.

'Back then, the locals were just learning to surf and not many tourists came. So I'd make everyone's surfboards. But now everybody wants the Australian shaper, because the pros ride them. With all the new shops and industry growing here, they have access to these boards now. They don't want a local board so I can't sell boards anymore.' He now has a job in the construction industry, but when Mundaka turns on, like everyone else in the area, he'll drop his tools and catch what he wants.

## PANTIN

Further west along the north coast of Spain, the coastline suddenly drops again to the south. Unlike many other countries, Spain's major cities are evenly dispersed inland and most towns by the ocean are small fishing villages, hugging the coasts and bays. One such place is Pantin. It's a beautiful coast to drive along and the air is different here. If your window is down you'll catch (if you're Australian) a familiar smell that refreshes your senses and invokes nostalgia. Looking around, you'll notice something else familiar — eucalyptus trees, and plenty of them, all the way to the beach. It is as if you'd woken up from a dream and landed on the east coast of Australia.

How they got there is an interesting story. Over 200 years ago, the First Fleet that had settled Australia was on its way back to England when it ran aground on these shores. The locals, accustomed to the ways of maritime hospitality, helped the English fix their vessels and gave them food and shelter. To repay that gesture, the English, amongst other things (there are quite a few red heads and blue eyes in these parts), gave the locals seeds from a eucalyptus tree. These trees are very dominant in their nature; they are also very thirsty and are often used to stabilise land. In Cuzco, for example, in the Andes, they were introduced to stop landslides; now they are everywhere. The same happened in Pantin. Eucalyptus trees have taken over the landscape, lining the hills and freshening the air.

The waves are good here too. Not many people surf them as most kids are into soccer. Between playing, working, drinking coffee in the town square and siestas, they do what Spanish people often do — sit on their balconies and watch the world go by. In this slower part of the world, they are world-champion observers of life. And in a place that couldn't be much further away from my own country, for one week of surfing, I never felt so at home.

## El MATADOR

Pablo Gutierrez is somewhere between the past, the present and the future of surfing in Spain. As he is one of the country's first professional surfers, his desire to compete has earned him the nickname of his country's symbol — the bullfighter, or 'el matador'. Born in Santander, the 26-year-old started surfing at a time when there was no surf industry and hardly any real surfers, so when Pablo told his parents he wanted to be a professional surfer, they were a little confused.

'I was a good soccer player when I was young. Surfing was not a big thing at all, so when I stopped playing soccer and started to surf, people couldn't believe it. There was only one surfboard company and it was hard to get the equipment. I would try to get secondhand boards from the pros, or from tourists, always pleading for a cheap price. Then I started to surf more, got some wins in the competition and started to make my career as a professional surfer,' Pablo explained. However, apart from the odd WQS event, there still weren't many surf events in Spain, as the country was much more interested in soccer.

'I started to travel to France. That's when I got a sponsorship from Rip Curl, because I won some events. This next year I will just do surf trips and the WQS. My life is good,' he continued.

These days, Pablo's parents better understand their son's life. He speaks fluent French, Spanish, Basque and English, travels the world and is leading a new generation of fiery Spaniards into the possibilities of life by the ocean.

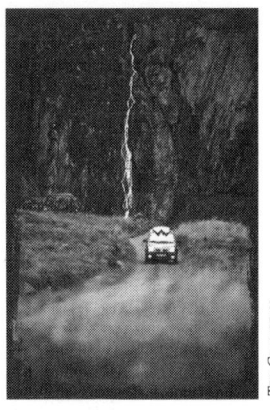

# NORDIC FRESH
## NORWAY ETC

Nathan Hedge and I were in Helsinki, Finland. With at least a week up our sleeve, and the longest leg of the tour looming, we thought we'd add some contrast to our lives. So we ventured almost as far away from the equator and coast as we could; somewhere between Europe and the Arctic Circle. We started in Helsinki, then travelled to Estonia and then drifted towards Germany; all places rich in both culture and history, but definitely lacking in surf culture. This was the prelude to our trip to Norway, where we would reunite with the ocean. Dreams of surfing beneath the fjords foretold a happy ending to our travels, but for now we were two fish out of water, trying to bring some balance to who we are and what we do.

While our attempt was initially to get away from surfing, we soon learned that surfing had actually beaten us to our destination. Like a slow moving tidal wave, surfing has made its way through waveless Europe, consuming consumers and furnishing dreams of a lifestyle around the ocean. We might have had other things to do in northern Europe, but it seemed northern Europe had plans for us too.

## FINLAND

'Wow! It's so good to come to a place where nobody knows you and you don't know anyone,' said Hog, regarding the peak hour traffic of the Finnish capital. A couple of surfers dragging big coffin bags caused the ladies with their finely designed handbags to stare. Their hands circled their hair for answers, and their questions were typical. 'What do you have in the bag — a boat?' I pretended it was the first time I'd heard the question. The busy scene was a change for Hog also. 'It's pretty levelling to not have someone to pick you up, with houses and cars ready. We're pretty spoilt, aren't we!' he laughed, appreciating the moment, as we dragged our boards all over the city looking for somewhere to stay.

We checked in to a local hotel and walked around the city. Everyone in Helsinki has blond hair and blue eyes, a melting pot of designer genes amongst ancient European architecture. They are all tall and beautiful; the women dress powerfully, the men dress attractively. Peak hour at any time is best observed, not participated in. We started drinking and watching, excited at the prospect of going out that night. As it was summer, the sun was still out, but in a few corners of the city, in the fading light, electricity beckoned with nighttime possibilities. People don't go out in the evening till about midnight in Helsinki. By that time, Heinekens and time had teamed up to ensure that our endeavours were useless.

Basically, we had become too drunk. We watched helplessly as all the hot girls walked in the opposite direction and made a mental note to ourselves: don't start drinking so early; go out later.

The next day we walked around again and did what most people do when travelling: checked out the art galleries and museums, then emailed our friends back home about our experiences abroad.

Only days earlier I had emailed my friend Corey O'Malley, a wordsmith and intellectual innovator. He read the dictionary for fun as a kid, hitchhiked around Australia as a teenager, clinically died for a few seconds on magic mushrooms in Mexico and maintains the only reason he wasn't repeatedly expelled from high school was 'because I kept winning against them computers in debating competitions'.

He should be writing books or delivering speeches to the UN or NATO, and maybe one day he will, but for now his bare feet are planted firmly amongst groups of hippies debating around fires in Africa, Indonesia, New Zealand and, during this week, Malawi.

'So, what do you know about Norway?' I asked in my email.

'I know an awful lot about Scandinavia. I know everything about Scandinavia. Of course, Scandinavia once ruled Europe. Not so very long ago. I also know what Scandinavia *isn't* — Finland. Finland is not actually considered to be part of Scandinavia as such. I know that. Scandinavia is Norway, Sweden, Denmark. That's the dual peninsula, and the three have very closely related languages. Finland — geographically, linguistically and culturally — is very different. So maybe one day you too can impress someone with this fact. Next time you hear someone mention Finland and Scandinavia in the same breath, murder them with the depth of your geo-knowledge. They won't believe you. It's a great fun and useless argument to have. And then when you go to "prove" it, some stupid website or seven will call Finland "Scandinavia".

'I also know that Norway shares a land border with Russia; strange, but true. Check it out. It's one of my very favourite land borders. I'd like to toboggan across it with Lapp reindeer herdsmen one day, whilst flying on mushrooms. They have perhaps the strongest magic mushrooms in the world in far northern Norway: big red ones, with white spots — very toxic! The Viking berserkers used to force-feed them to captives then drink their (that is, the captives') piss. The captives' bodies would filter out the toxins and leave the hallucinogens in the urine. The captives would die. The warriors would quite literally drink piss, trip hard and hack monks to pieces.

'I also know that according to my taste Norway has the ugliest women in Scandinavia. Their slightly pinched faces must be as a result of those blasting North Atlantic winds. Not like the gentle Baltic breezes that give that kiss of angelic zesty Nordic vigour to those statuesque Danes and Swedes. Best of all, I know that if you get above the Arctic Circle before the 21 September equinox, you will see the true midnight sun. It won't set. You might even see the aurora borealis …'

## ESTONIA

Our plan had changed. We would cross the Baltic Sea to Estonia in the old USSR, and then make our move to Norway. We boarded a boat, not unlike the one we had sailed on a month earlier during a Search trip in Indonesia. But unlike on that trip, this time cold winds lashed the Baltic, and the sea was like an island in an ocean of landmass. The team — Mick Fanning, Benny Dunn, Raoni Monteiro and Knoxy — wasn't with us this time and we were wearing jeans and jumpers instead of board shorts. Also, instead of coffin bags full of surfboards, boardies and sunscreen, all we had were our backpacks.

When we arrived, it was clear it wasn't a holiday destination. In fact, I'm sure not many people know it exists, let alone where it is on a map. We were in Tallinn, Estonia's capital, and it was interesting to see how a part of the former USSR was trying to catch up with the rest of the world in an economic and fashion sense. We basically spent our time people watching. Nobody in Tallinn knew what surfing was, let alone had felt the rush of moving water. They played soccer, studied, worked in the markets; they did whatever it took to press fast forward on their lives and achieve a lifestyle like they had seen on TV.

These former Eastern Bloc countries have only recently emerged from the Soviet grip. To give a little history, Estonia was occupied by the Soviet Union in June 1940, after Stalin and Hitler's agreement to divide Eastern Europe into 'spheres of Special Interest'. Hitler, being who he was, took back control of the country and the Nazis occupied Estonia from 1941 to 1944, sapping its resources to continue their war effort. The Soviets regained it in 1944 and when Communist Russia began to fall apart in 1991, the Eastern Bloc countries under the 'Iron Curtain' made the push for independence, which was finally achieved in 1994.

The wounds are still fresh, especially in the older generation. They wear grey clothes and purposefully live practised lives of inconspicuousness. Under Soviet rule, any creative idea, thought or mode of dress was crushed with an iron fist, so they still wear things, say things and do things that keep them from standing out.

However, the generation that has grown up since 1991 is heading in a different direction. But while they are adding colour and opportunity, there is still a lot of grey to grow out of — like the green growing out of a burnt tree.

It was time to adjust the pH levels and get in the salt, so off we went to Norway, armed with information and inspiration. But there was one more stopover, at a place that is surf crazy. It is a place where they know everything about surfing, they even have everything — except waves.

## GERMANY

When you walk through the streets of Berlin you can actually see its history very clearly. On one side of the city the buildings are quite methodical and grey; the other side is colourful, creative and expressionistic. Between them, a line was once drawn between east and west, communism and capitalism — and it remained for twenty-seven years between 1961 and 1989. I spoke to a woman who was on the wrong side of the wall when it was constructed — she didn't see her husband for twenty-seven years. It was quite ridiculous to think that something like this could happen in modern times.

These days, Germany is full of colour. The country is a world economic leader and the people wear their riches well. The population is smart, very well educated, multi-lingual and wealthy. This creates great opportunities for their youth who have an exuberant appetite for experience — and part of that energy is directed towards surfing. Believe it or not, Germany is surf crazy. They have professional surfers, surf shops, and magazines.

*Surf Europe* editor Paul Evans explained: 'Well, they're the most motivated and well-resourced surf nation of eighty million people — but without a true surf coast. Germans have spread their wings south and westward particularly, with German surf camps and surf schools lining some of Europe's finest surf coasts in Portugal, as well as maintaining strongholds on the southwest coast of France, the Canaries and further afield in Costa Rica.

'Some of the earlier German migrants to warmer European shores are now fathers to Europe's finest young pros like Marlon Lipke [recently the first German to compete in a WCT] and Nicholaus Von Rupp, seventeen-year-old runner-up in the Portuguese men's national titles. Both are German nationals who were raised in southern Portugal, and are sponsored by big multinationals like Lufthansa and X-Markets. Meanwhile, on the industry side, the snowboard business based in alpine Germany and their Deutsche-tongued neighbour, Austria, continues to power Europe's "freesport" industry.'

I know one German surfer. He has fashioned himself a job where he can do what he can't do at home — surf. He travels around, commentating WCT events for the German web audience, translating articles for German surf mags and doing whatever else he can to satisfy his love of surfing.

His name is Quirin Rohleder and I caught up with him to discover more about surfing in Germany.

'Surfing is booming in Germany. More and more people are doing it. The main thing is that Germans have a lot of spending power, which means they travel a lot. Another important fact is the lifestyle. Everyone wants to live it. You shouldn't forget, though, that the majority of people in Germany have no idea about surfing and that for most people surfing is still windsurfing. However, it's also not true that you can't surf here. Germany has a bit of coastline and people have been surfing in Germany since the sixties, mainly on the island of Sylt. And even where there's no sea, there is the river. Lots of people living in Munich get in contact with surfing through the river wave. Actually, there are two river waves in Munich; these are standing waves.

'Then there's snowboarding. A lot of people spend their winter holidays in the mountains. So for people who got into snowboarding, it is sort of a natural transition to go surfing in summer.

'There aren't many Germans who get into contact with surfing early on in their lives, because surfing means travelling, and travelling means that you need to be a bit older. I started a bit earlier, which meant my life evolved around my holidays. During school, I would work and save up money to be able to spend time at the beach in my holidays. The first stop for most Germans is obviously France; for me it was Italy in winter — Varazze — a good spot about seven hours away from Munich.

'Students are better off. They have three months of holidays at a time and many of them travel extensively. And as soon as you work, well, it's pretty much over. All you have then are the two weeks in summer and the two weeks in winter, which is really hard because you always need at least one week to sort of get back into it.'

## NORWAY

Hog and I had spent the last week or more in cities and we craved more natural surroundings.

The thing that captivated my attention more than anything else in Norway was the fjords. Surfing beneath them was something I really wanted to experience, but we had to move quickly. We needed to be in Trestles in four days for the next event on the WCT Tour, so we arrived in Oslo with a purpose.

We stayed at a mutual friend's place in the city. It belonged to an Australian rich boy who was working at his own designing business by day and sailing yachts by week's end. Trophies and photos on the wall confirmed his stories and the can of VB on the windowsill reminded him of his roots — and appealed to our homesickness. He had built his own little Australia in his one-bedroom apartment.

We went straight out for a party, as you do. The first thing we noticed was a hole burning in our pockets. For example, after a five-minute taxi ride and four beers at a local nightclub, we were down about US$200. And we hadn't even had our second beer!

But the girls were amazing. Unlike Corey, Hog and I were calling it the best place on earth for natural beauties.

The next morning we woke up, walked around the city, worked the Internet cafe circuit and met some girls from the night before.

'You should see up north,' a local lady had said. 'Imagine the mountains of New Zealand coming down to the coast. It's very rugged and beautiful.' She was talking about the fjords. 'And just off the coast, in between north Atlantic fronts, you will see some great waves. But it takes you a while to get there and you need to be there a week at least to appreciate it, because it can be bad weather.'

A check with the weather bureau confirmed cloud cover for a week up north and the swell was small. But Trestles was expecting some swell. So like that, the decision was made to leave. We had spent all our money and experienced some culture, as far away from the beach as possible. But my yearning for the fjords still tugged at me. I hoped one day to return — to surf beneath them, riding the northern seas like a wild Viking. It is a wish that has not yet been fulfilled.

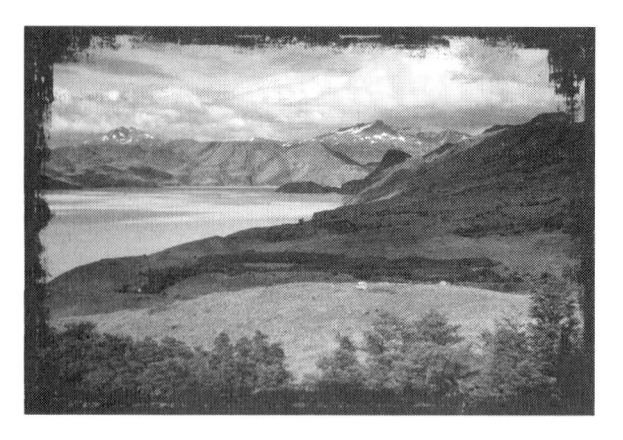

# CORRIDOR OF CONTRAST
## CHILE

I do not hold prejudice against any animal, but it is a plain fact that the turkey vulture is not served well by its appearance. They hover with menace and suggestion in the sea mist complaining about death, yet looking for it at the same time. On the Chilean coastline, the driest coast in the world, they don't have to look far. It is all around them. There is no grass to eat, no shrubs to hide behind and no rivers to drink from. Just desert sand and rock; lifeless, colourless, almost odourless. The only smell in the air is from salt, or from the odd carcass and droppings of birds. That's the life cycle on the northern coast of Chile: desert eats animal, turkey vultures pick at the carcass — simple, lifeless, colourless. The ocean is also monotonic, reflecting the constant grey fog that soars with the vultures. At times it's hard to tell where the sky meets the horizon — and the sea birds also have trouble, losing themselves in the grey, camouflaged into dullness. The locals say that when God finished making the world, he put the leftover stuff here. He didn't have much left over.

# THE LUNAR COAST

I was in Chile, looking at a lunar landscape, surfing ledgey waves, eating fish and limbering my Spanish tongue. I had a week up my sleeve before the second instalment of Rip Curl's Search WCT landed in Arica on the north coast. The first thing I noticed was this: Chile has some interesting geography. It's sandwiched between one of the world's greatest mountain ranges — the Andes — and the world's greatest ocean — the Pacific. The Andes run parallel to the coastline, bordering an incredibly narrow corridor of land which is less than 100 kilometres in some areas. This is rare; picture it in the back of your mind. In defiance of its barren nature, some of the most colourful cultures, including the Incas, have evolved here, borrowing from all of nature's extremes. Their story is one of triumph and mystery.

But in the south, the coastline is not all as lifeless as the north. South of Santiago, the landscape defiantly starts to become green, as though the glaciers and high-mountain peaks of the Andes could no longer deny it sustenance. Animals and life come back, combining with a boiling marine life and waves aplenty.

This part of the Pacific Ocean is also very interesting and has a plethora of pelagic activity which would excite any marine biologist. Anchovies are as abundant as the salt they swim in, supplying protein to the raging population of marine birds that swoop upon them with practised skill, bombing the water by the thousands.

Put simply, the Andean mountains do what they do best — they climb. The ocean does what it does best — it swells. And the 6435 kilometres of coastline is reaping some interesting benefits. In fact, this place is so unique, it has basically created its own weather system.

# PATTERNS

When humans have time on their hands they become curious. This inquisitiveness is often lost in our modern-day BlackBerry agendas and economic activities. But travelling gives us time to ask questions. Fingers used to fondling phones can find a global map in the back of an in-flight magazine and wonder what Moscow looks like. Spending time on the desert coast of Chile, you ask a lot of questions. My questions started with why is it so hot on land here, but so cold in the water? This led to: why — even at tropical latitudes — does the western coast of almost every continent feature a desert bordered by cold water? Picture them: Australia, South America and Africa — even Hawaii. My initial idle observation started to become an obsession. I needed an explanation and, as fate would have it, someone showed up. Enter James Dell, a quantitative marine scientist from Tasmania who contributes marine and atmospheric research to the CSIRO. I met him in J-Bay when I was writing this story, and he made sense of the question that was starting to debilitate me.

'The presence of cold ocean currents along the continent's western side is a big reason,' he said. 'These currents arrive at the coast via what is called the deep ocean conveyor system. These deep ocean currents carry very cold and nutrient-rich waters that have travelled great distances, north and east, across the ocean floor, originating from the southern ocean near to the Antarctic continent. Once these deep currents hit the coasts of Chile and southern Peru they have nowhere to go but up, bringing cold, dark water to the surface of the ocean, which affects both air temperatures and precipitation (mostly as fog) along the Pacific coast.

'The fog forms off the coast as a result of moist oceanic air moving in over the cold coastal water, and condensing. It sucks all the moisture out of the ground, forming the desert. As the mist reaches the land it hits hot air again and evaporates, forming what the Chileans call "Garua", which is a bizarre super fine mist. A similar system is found on Namibia's Skeleton Coast on the southwest coast of Africa, where the same combination of desert, cold ocean and mountains combine.'

## FRANCISCO

The Incas were a strange culture. I was in Africa and was spending my time in between surfs reading about them. From the restrictive altitudes in the Andes where they were born, to the barren deserts of the Peruvian and Chilean coast, they more or less dominated most of South America between the twelfth and fourteenth century.

Nothing much has changed for the Chileans of today. To succeed, they must first do battle with the landscape. This struggle is ongoing and realising it cannot be won is the first step. As the Incas demonstrated with their irrigation systems, first the environment must be understood and then tamed for advantage. Added to the harsh environment is a struggling economy in which most people don't have enough money to buy a schoolbook, let alone afford a teacher. In this country there is little access to good education or well-paying jobs. For Chilean surfers, the obstacles on the path to professionalism are as high as the Andes themselves. But some are having a go.

Francisco is a 25-year-old professional surfer from Chile. I met him during the Rip Curl Search WCT in Arica, where he had come to buy one of the twenty-seven boards Mick Fanning had left behind. Not knowing exactly what to expect, and knowing how many boards break,

Mick had shipped thirty-five surfboards to Chile for this event. The excitement on Francisco's face betrayed his need for a bargain. 'Can I have these seven?' he asked. 'For one thousand?' The availability of good surfboards is not something Chilean surfers are used to, and as there was a queue of eager buyers, he had to move swiftly to claim the foreign booty.

Francisco lives in Santiago, where most of the surf industry is based and where the events are held, but he also makes regular journeys to the south coast.

'There are some good waves there and not many surfers,' he said. 'In Santiago we have mostly beach breaks. This is where we have the competitions and the sponsors so it is important to be here. But down south we have perfect point breaks. I love going down there. No people around; beautiful country and beautiful waves.' His smile backed up the claim and you could see his eyes searching the back of his brain for fond memories of empty line-ups and green headlands. 'But the water is even colder down there; you have to wear 4/3 plus booties, sometimes even more.'

Although he is sponsored, Francisco earns a modest amount, even by Chilean standards. It is probably just enough to pay for his entry fees and for the petrol to get to the competitions. He moves up and down the coast looking for waves and competing in the national competitions. But not everyone has that luxury. Chile is a Third World country and the flow of equipment and money is as dry as the coastline. The surfers buy boards off tourists, learn how to fix broken and failing boards, and make their way from the shore breaks to outside reefs and points — and finally to competition.

As Chilean surfers are so isolated, the only link to the outside world used to come from whatever DVDs tourists had left behind, which showed them a level of surfing they didn't know existed. But with the advent of internet accessibility, Chileans are seeing pros on a daily basis now, and so their standard is improving as they have access to more equipment and inspiration. Globalisation means we will see more surfers from interesting places in years to come, maybe even from Chile? 'I hope so,' Francisco said. 'We have a long way to go, but we try hard to make a life as a professional surfer.'

Francisco is lucky as he comes from a wealthy family and is thus not dependent on the fledgling national surfing economy. But he also, like most of his peers, dreams of one day seeing a Chilean reach the world stage in surfing. 'The [national] tour is growing here and we have some prize money and good surfers,' he said. 'I hope one day we can be on the World Tour.'

## HISTORY

Let's backtrack a little and get really clear on what Chile is. About 10,000 years ago, migrating Native Americans settled in fertile valleys along the coast of what is now Chile. The Incas briefly extended their empire into what is now northern Chile, but the area's barrenness prevented extensive settlement. Europeans reached Chile when Diego de Almagro and his band of Spanish conquistadors entered the country from Peru in 1535, seeking gold. The Spanish encountered hundreds of thousands of Native Americans from various cultures in the area that modern Chile now occupies. The conquest of Chile began in earnest in 1540 and was carried out by Pedro de Valdivia, one of Spanish explorer Francisco Pizarro's lieutenants, who founded the city of Santiago on 12 February 1541. Although the Spanish did not find the extensive deposits of gold and silver they sought, there was one thing they didn't check — the surf.

The fact that the country is narrow suits the surfer perfectly, craving only coastline and a steep gradient to cause waves to break. Chile has both. Its position is in prime Pacific real estate — that entire ocean, all that coastline, all those possibilities … However, it took a while for surfing to get started in Chile. The first local surfing dates from the beginning of the seventies, but it has really only been in the last few years that the international spotlight has shed its light on the consistency of the surf, the infinity of good locations and the huge perfect waves with no one surfing them.

The local charge is now being led by three of the best Chilean surfers: Ramón Navarro and Cristian Merello — local big wave chargers from Pichilemu — and Diego Medina, winner of the 2005 Billabong XXL Paddle Award for a monster caught at Punta de Lobos. A solid Chilean scene is starting to emerge and grow at a rapid pace.

The country can be separated into roughly three big regions. The north, with the driest desert in the world and its rocky bottoms, produces some of Chile's most powerful and hollow waves. The central region, which is the most accessible due to its proximity to Santiago, has many spots that are for the most part friendly, but which sometimes see fifteen to twenty foot days. Then there is the southern region, a pristine green environment overlooking a string of left tubing point breaks just waiting to be explored. With a national average of 300 days a year of surf, it is very unlikely that Chile will have a long flat spell. Swells hit the coast of Chile year round and they can hit hard.

It was these elements that led Rip Curl to bring their Search WCT here — and thus the reason I was in Arica. The team had arrived, the banners were planted, the scaffold was being erected, and the 600mm lenses were arriving along with the quiver of surfboards in the back of trucks. The circus had arrived — and things might never be the same again.

## SEARCHING FOR MOUNTAINS AND SLABS

'We came to Chile because it offered some fresh experiences for the ASP World Tour,' said Neil Ridgway, our group advertising and marketing chairman. 'It presented a new culture and a new wave that would challenge the world's best.'

Everyone on tour loves this event because in a repetitious tour life, it enables them to break the monotony and go somewhere different every year. Since unique destinations are chosen, it also rules out the use of local knowledge and places everyone on a level playing field as far as wave knowledge and selection goes. Arica in Chile was about as different as you could get.

'This place looks like Mars,' said Pancho Sullivan, regarding the surrounding landscape. I had just picked him up from the airport and we were making our way to the event site. Around us was red dirt, its texture decided by either rocks or sand of the same colour. The Andes start their climb early here, but that doesn't alter the landscape; it's all just red and very lunar-like.

Soon we were driving adjacent to the ocean. A long beach made its way out to a little harbour, and finally to an island that sat beneath a menacing cliff. Pancho looked over the island, where El Gringo's breaks. It is a serious wave. 'Fuck, this is it!' said Pancho. 'It looks like a wave for bodyboarders.' The wave breaks very close to the rocks with a lot of power. Quite simply, it's a very scary and challenging wave. But it is also very short; you come out of the barrel next to the dry reef.

'It's going to be a challenge for the tour, huh?' said Andy Higgins, Search WCT Director. 'It will be interesting to see how they handle this wave because I don't think anyone has surfed it to the level it can be surfed yet.' It was a true statement, and while we studied the water intently, we soon realised there was only one way to get the good waves — go for everything and find out.

'I knew I had to just go for everything,' said Mick Fanning after his first surf. 'Lefts, rights, big ones, small ones. We're going to have to attack this wave. Just keep catching waves and pull in looking for good ones.'

And so the surfers did. Boards were broken, blood was spilt, heads were concussed — and some amazing surfing was done.

In one heat, Andy Irons got two 9s in the first five minutes of his thirty-five-minute heat and then came in. 'It's too fucking cold out there,' he said, back in the competitors' area.

Andy came in with twenty-seven minutes to go. He literally could have been back home in the shower when the hooter went — and still won. Andy would go on to win the event, as he does in these sorts of waves.

One day the surf picked up and we surfed El Bommie, which is the premier big wave destination in Chile. It was around fifteen feet and like a mini Waimea Bay. Kelly was the standout. While we were all survival stancing the big drops, Kelly was taking off late and attempting the barrel. He always finds a way to be better than the rest.

When we partied at the end of the event at a local's house, something very rare happened — it rained, although it almost seemed as if it was the fog that was crying.

'My God, the first time it has ever rained in Chile — and you are here. You are lucky to see this,' exclaimed our host.

## JESSE

You don't have to drive far to break the monotony of the desert coast in Chile. Within an hour you can be inland in the mountains, looking at rich glaciers 4000 metres above sea level; or, just south of Santiago, you come to a series of point breaks that has become famous amongst travelling surfers. For most Chileans, contrast is a one-hour drive, but for Jesse Fean, former ASP media manager, it's a short flight.

'I first found out about Chile through Derek Hynd,' said Jesse, who now works for Insight in LA. 'I guess he was involved with Rip Curl at the time and doing some research on new places and he found this spot south of Santiago where there were a bunch of good point breaks. He had bought some land there. It was something that I always wanted to do — have somewhere to escape to, learn another language and get into another culture. At the time I was doing the tour and I needed a place to get away from everything. The place sounded fascinating. I probably wouldn't have done it if I had seen it, so the mystery trapped me too.

'Derek rang me and told me there was a block of land for sale next door to him. I'd never been there — never even seen it — and I bought it. It cost me US$20,000. That was in 2000. I ended up going there and loving the place. In Santiago the people are into business, money and the fast life, but if you drive a few hours down the coast, all of a sudden the desert transforms into lush rolling green hills, with headlands around every corner. The Andes are right there — it's one of the most stunning places you'll ever see. The people there lead a really simple life. Their whole focus is on spending quality time with family and friends, talking and being simple. They go out and catch their fish and that's all they need to worry about — feeding themselves and their family — and they are happy. It's such a nice place to escape to and tap into that relaxed energy.

'I go there a few times a year; I've built a house on my block of land. I spent a lot of money building and setting up the house, but you can't put a price on what I experience there. For example, I fly there for Christmas and spend two weeks with my next-door neighbour and his family. I love how they approach life and they feel like my family now too. They are amazing people with an amazing way of life.'

He paused and then showed me the other side. 'Well, the water's cold. And it's a lot of work to get there and set up, because no matter where you come from, it's hard. It's not as cheap as you'd expect and the waves aren't always perfect. But to tell the truth, I've had some of the best waves and best times of my life in Chile.'

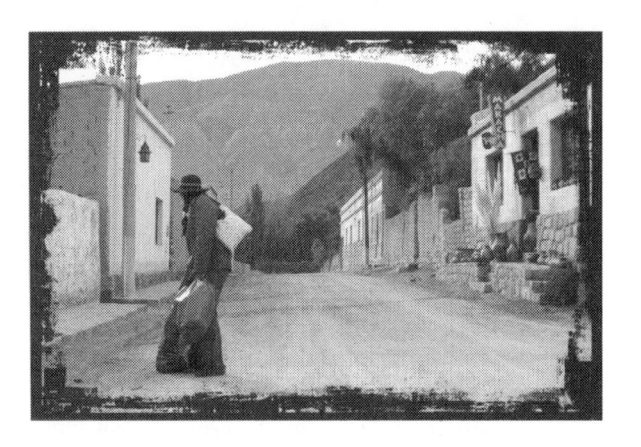

# BUENOS DIAS
## ARGENTINA

There are some things in life we know. For example, the earth is round; the speed of light is 300,000 kilometres per second; in a good life you'll live 650,000 hours — and if you fall off on a dry reef, it hurts. And there are some things we suppose, tinker with and hypothesise — like the number of stars in the sky and the reason God put flies on earth. Some things we see, experience, feel and touch; some things we just believe because a scientist said so.

Such issues are often thought of in Argentina. Since university is free and jobs are rare, the Argentinians have become a nation of thinkers. They study — and keep on studying until they find a job. Since this can take a while — often a lifetime — they keep studying. They have become a bit top heavy in their wealth: boasting a brain full of ideas, but empty in the back pocket of the fuel to further their passionate dreams. They love and live the beach, but when I arrived, there were some other things going on.

## ARGENTINA

I was in Buenos Aires early in 2001. A man was walking across the street, holding his son's hand. They looked into the rubbish bin, inspected some old food and plastic bottles, took anything of worth and moved on to the next bin. There was little activity; rubbish blew through the streets like tumbleweed. What is usually known as the Paris of South America was semi-deserted. Even the protesters and thieves had given up. There was nobody there to hear them and nothing left to steal. Three hundred thousand people had left the country, five different presidents had taken office in five days, the value of the peso had dropped by 75 per cent, there were riots, strikes, and fear, and 50 per cent of the population had fallen below the poverty line. I went to an ATM; it was not dispensing cash — all money was frozen. I walked around the streets bewildered. I'd never seen anything like this. Only one in five shops were open. The ones that weren't had been turned into fortresses to protect against thieves.

'It's so hard for the families,' said Jose, a girl I had met during a previous trip in Peru. She had big brown eyes that took in the scenes of her city, trying to understand, trying to explain to someone like me without understanding it herself. Borrowing her mum's car and caring nature, she drove me around, explaining the situation.

'The families have worked all their life to save money. Maybe they have saved enough to have a holiday, to start a business or send their kids overseas to work and travel. Now that money will buy them food for one week. It is horrible.'

The city is beautiful in its architecture, both romantic and historic. It is almost as if you have arrived in Barcelona, or another big European city of cultural infinities. I imagined the Latino dance classes; the universities spilling into local bars; the older generation watching the world go by while sipping short blacks on street corners.

In a city of thinkers, they were now familiar with a new word — economics. I don't know whether the situation had been caused by corruption, like in other South American cities, or whether the powers-that-be just fucked up. I remembered that father looking through bins with his son, other families begging for money.

It was a weird thing to come into contact with, and lent perspective to what we call hard times. I needed to get to a place where wealth is in the experience, or you could at least escape momentarily from the problems associated with big cities and their economics. A place where wealth is decided by storms 1000 kilometres away and the weather overhead.

I don't want to give any false impressions. You are not going to get barrelled in Argentina. You won't ride the biggest, longest or best waves of your life; that will just not happen. There are over thirty surf spots in the Mar del Plata region alone, but you won't find great surfers. You'll get warm weather for the most part; warm water and enough waves to satisfy a surf. But I'll tell you something — it's a happening little town. There are nightclubs, hot girls, parties. I found myself there for a WQS. The wind swell that came up for the event may as well have been in a small bay; it was barely breaking. So, being young and stupid, we went out every night. Their nightclubs had skateboard ramps and hot girls behind the bars. They knew why people were coming and they catered for it. One such nightclub was three storeys high and full of beautiful women. What is it with South America and the ratio of women to men?

The name in Latin — *argentum* — means silver, and since the Spanish set up here in 1516, this country has experienced an influx and outflux of people. 'During World War II, a lot of Nazis escaped here,' a local told me. Behind dark lenses, eighty-year-old men and their offspring still looked like they were hiding. They enjoyed the beach and watching the surfers, but crime still tinkered in their mind; you could feel it. 'It meant a lot of crooks came here, so it can be dangerous at times and you need to be aware. But most people are good Catholic people — and the few that aren't just want to have fun and party.'

We surfed a few times in and around heats, but it was terrible. The ASP has since banned organisers putting on an event above a four star because they just don't have the wave quality. It was a good decision. But it's a shame that the surfing world doesn't come to Mar del Plata anymore, because it's hard for them to go to the world, especially during this time. Still there was that passion for life you can't deny. It's contagious and unreal to be around.

Argentina has a weird mix of people — escaped Nazis, the rare Indian, the Spanish Conquistadors and a massive youth population with a wealth of knowledge trying to figure it all out. It's like it's trying too hard to be European in culture and American in ways of finance. However, I thought it was pretty cool.

I'll tell you what else Argentina is good at: meat. You will find the best steaks here, often in carveries where you will have the opportunity to eat every piece of the cow. After my trip to Argentina, I participated in a social experiment. I became a vegiquarium, which I defined as eating vegetables and anything out of the ocean. When I stopped over for a night in Buenos Aires, I dutifully devoured every piece of the cow in case I needed to store the protein for the year of my insanity.

That same night, some girls had taken us out and were theorising on economics, on how to fix the problems of the world, starting with

Argentina. They were smart and beautiful, with the passion innate to every Latino. Soon they would be in charge — somehow — of their country's future. As I write this seven years down the track I wonder where they're at now. Argentina has returned to a semi-strong and functioning economy. The people are coming back and the number of fathers begging for money on the streets is normal for a big city. I wondered if those girls had anything to do with it.

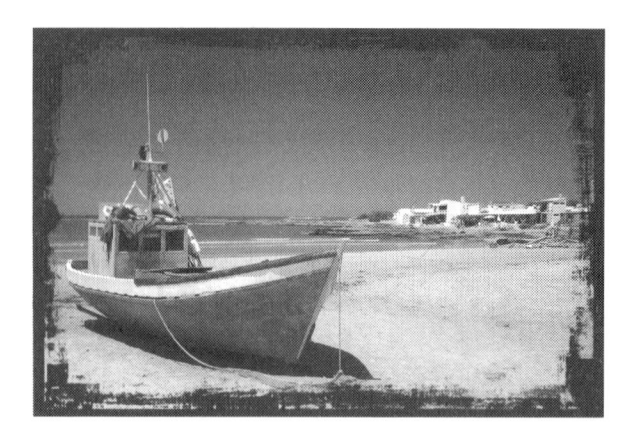

# MEAT IN THE SANDWICH
## URUGUAY

I don't know how they still supposed the earth was flat when the Spanish ships dipped over the horizon in the sixteenth century to discover the New World. It really wasn't that long ago in the scheme of things, but the journeys of those days were partly to prove that the world was in fact a sphere — as well as to bring home precious raw materials and slaves.

It was not a new idea that the earth is round. Ptolemy produced a map of a globular earth as early as AD140; the Egyptians knew it; and the idea was documented in the greatest library in the world in Alexandria. However, the notion contradicted the interpretation of the Bible so the church rejected the idea, calling it heresy. So the library — like anything that contradicted the Bible, humans included — was burnt. Of course the earth was flat — everyone could see that! Above the Earth was Heaven and below the Earth was Hell, and in between lived Man and Woman — that was the Bible's idea.

Now, a flat earth is fine, unless you want to go to sea. The problem for sailors is that if the Earth is flat, then it must have edges. And if it has edges, then boats can fall off them. And if your boat falls off the edge of the world, well — you get the point. So for many years, sailors lived in fear of losing sight of land, and sea voyagers hugged the coastlines. But during the fourteenth, fifteenth and sixteenth centuries exploration of the oceans of the world began in earnest and islands, countries and continents were discovered. One of them was Uruguay. There, the adventurers found gold, much of which is still unmined to this day.

They say that the further you go south in Brazil, the better the women get. It is not by accident that just to the south of Brazil is a little country called Uruguay. Like in Brazil, the small population of 3.3 million people that live in Uruguay are mostly females. I have no idea why this happens, but their beauty is a fact which you can see the truth of on every beach and in every nightclub in South America. These women are everywhere, lying on the beaches, exposing their bodies to the omnipresent sun. They live with passion and energy, but at the same time know how to relax.

Even on a map, there's something that looks cool about Uruguay. And when you go there, there is something even cooler. I landed there in 1998, in its capital, Montevideo. While all roads seem to head towards its capital, all residents head to the beaches in the summer months, enjoying a long and beautiful coastline from the Atlantic border with Brazil, down to the mouth of the Rio de la Plata, and upriver to the border of Argentina. Punta del Este is the place most people go, and the place that I went for a WQS.

It seemed a lot more affluent than Brazil or Argentina. Not many people surfed, but everyone lived for the beach. It was there that I was introduced to coffee. I remember the feeling hitting me and having to go for a run before my heat to settle the shakes. They drink coffee like water there and I guess this contributes to their endless energy. There weren't very many surfers, mainly because there weren't many people. The majority live in its capital and play soccer. The beach is only somewhere they go on the weekends or on holidays.

Because there are no mountains of note in the country, there tends to be a lot of wind. It is generally welcome to the people sunbaking on the beach, but to surfers, it means wind-blown conditions by lunchtime on most days. This also causes wind swells, so like in Brazil and Argentina, you can get some fun beach breaks, but mostly the surf is weak and junky. The waves we had for the event were okay. My memory tells me Greg Emslie won it. But I'll never forget the fashion parade — the reef bikini models battling it out to be Miss Reef, to have the honour of displaying their body in glossy magazines and being whistled at. Bums are the pride of this part of the world and the girls spend a lot of their time training or tanning them. It's pretty cool and a good place to go if you're looking for that kind of thing.

There hasn't been another surf event there since I went in '98. Also, there has been nothing of world attention, no news of rising sports stars, of mass murders or anything else that makes news headlines. And so Uruguay has remained a little secret of particular gems — a place to party, to meet girls and share the beach lifestyle.

Uruguay was discovered in 1516, a short time after Magellan circumnavigated the globe in 1522, thus proving that the world was round. I wonder if the waves and beautiful beaches will be off the edge of most people's maps for much longer.

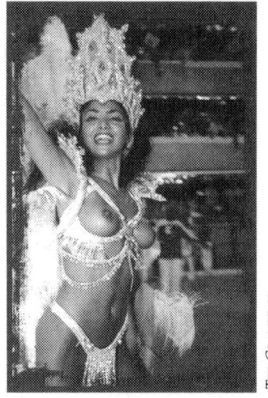

# JUNGLE BOOTY
## BRAZIL

BLEEDING all over the floor of his own home, the number one on the World Qualifying Series couldn't believe he was about to die. His hands were tied behind his back and blood oozed from a puncture wound in his side where he had just been stabbed.

Earlier that day, he had held a trophy above his head for winning the first event of the tour. Life was good — but now it couldn't have been worse. Two men had broken into his apartment, beaten him and his wife, robbed them and now, dissatisfied with their spoils, held a gun to their heads. 'We are going to fucking kill you,' they yelled in Portuguese. They had robbed him of his prize money, his possessions — and his blood, which continued to drain alarmingly into a pool of dark red. And now they promised to finish him off and burn his body if he didn't give them what they wanted. 'We want euro,' they kept saying. 'Give me or I fucking kill you!'

Jean de Silva, one of Brazil's leading surfers, had tears in the corners of his eyes as he recalled the story. 'They had taken my laptop, some clothes … I didn't have any euro, but I had some US dollars. At that moment, that was all I had. They took everything of mine. I said, "Take it, please — anything." I thought for sure they were going to kill me, because I had seen their faces. I was tied up and just waiting to die …'

Jean de Silva had just won US$10,000 — and, in the same day, lost it all. 'I guess my name was in the papers so the robbers knew I'd have something,' he reflected. Jean was robbed and almost shot; he was left bleeding, tied up along with his wife, his possessions gone.

'Did you tell the police?' I asked.

'No way! They would kill me! I still have my life — and I am stoked for that.'

In Brazil, the things that are given to you can be taken away again so easily. The people of Brazil live in a country of uncertainty, but it is this precariousness that gives birth to their passion to live every day and every second as if it were their last — a passion for life that is unrivalled and extremely contagious.

## JUNGLE BOOTY

Anyone with an appetite for surfing may be lured by the 9687 kilometres of Atlantic coastline and the sunny weather, the parties and festivals, the golden beaches and beautiful bodies that line it. But Brazil is interesting for so much more. Occupying more than half the continent, it is the largest country in South America in both area and population. In fact, it has more people than all the other countries in South America combined. The mighty Amazon — the world's second-longest, though largest, river — dominates the north, cut by the equator. Brazil also has an extensive logging industry which rapes the world's greatest rainforest at a rate of a football field a second, creating land for cattle grazing to supply Big Macs and Whoppers to the world's obese. (The Amazon Basin is about the size of France and 14 per cent of its trees have been cut down since 1970.)

More than anything, Brazilians live and breathe beach culture, so much so that 80 per cent of all Brazilian residents live within 320 kilometres of its shores. They are all about the beach. The nation's capital, Brasilia, was built 970 kilometres inland in an effort to attract people deeper into the jungle that is Brazil. It didn't really work.

## JESUS CHRIST

Images of the Big Man, standing tall above the world's most vibrant city, are enough to bring anyone to the carnival city of Rio de Janeiro. Cloaked in his best cement robe and standing tall like a proud father, the statue of Jesus Christ watches with quiet confidence over the endless mountains that climb and fall into bays, valleys and finally, the sea — one of his best pieces of work. From this vantage point, there is no city in the world as picturesque. Bays of blue water exit the ocean and wrap around lush green mountains and pockets of city infrastructure. The Rio coastline faces east into the Atlantic like a generously proportioned set of breasts above a tucked-in stomach. It also creates a lot of ocean swell.

Locals would have you believe that surfing in Brazil started there in Rio (it actually began in Sao Paulo in 1938). While the world has only felt the impact of Brazilian surfers in recent years, the beach culture in Brazil ranks as one of the world's strongest. 'Nobody likes to work in Rio,' said Paulo Mauro, a Brazilian pro surfer. 'They all want to go to the beach.' You don't need to be a rocket scientist to work that one out. The long sandy beaches are littered with volleyball nets, soccer fields, exercise equipment and more thongs (G-strings) than you'll see anywhere else in the world. Everyone wears G-strings in Brazil: fat, thin, old, young. Of course, this isn't always a great thing, but more often than not, it is, because everyone respects their bodies and their health so much. And everything you hear about beautiful Brazilian women, believe it!

'I can't believe Australian girls get fat,' said Sebastian Rojas, a surf photographer from Brazil. 'Don't they want to take care of their bodies?' He was genuinely puzzled. In Brazil, the female population greatly outweighs the male population, only in numbers, of course, so they have to present well or face the dreaded situation of being left on the shelf. So what happens is a role reversal — the women chase the man. It's epic! Above all, Rio is a fun city that has it all. But while ritzy buildings line the shores of beautiful beaches, *favelas* (slums) lurk in the background, depressing scars of a Third World country. From his high-up perch, looking at these slums hiding between the expensive suburbs, Jesus Christ must wonder where along the line the country went wrong.

## SAO PAULO

Flying into Sao Paulo International Airport, the contradictions are endless. Even before the captain announced our descent, the view was amazing. As far as the eye could see were buildings, built around buildings built on top of buildings — a concrete jungle with a halo of smog climbing like a chimney over the second most populated city in the world (New Delhi is the first). I'm told that an upright human's uninterrupted view to the horizon is 11 kilometres. From 10,000 feet, the horizon must be pretty far away. As I flew in, all I could see was this treeless and greenless concrete jungle for hundreds of kilometres. Modern buildings share the rising dust with *favelas*; however, like their residents, they never mingle. There is no middle class here. There are few if any trees and any sign of human life is swallowed by the sheer enormity of the built environment. The buildings continue to the horizon; every now and then the monotony is broken by a group of high-rises, or higher-rises, then *favelas*, then high-rises and higher-rises.

But one thing was missing from this picture: the stuff they use to build their concrete and the stuff they use to escape from it; the thing that is in Brazilian culture as much as the passion is in their blood — the sand of the beaches.

'I live in Sao Paulo,' said Renan Rocha, former top ten surfer and one of the longest standing Brazilian professional surfers. 'But I have a beach house as well. I spend Monday to Thursday in the city, because you just have to. Everything is there. Business, shops, restaurants, office. If you want to do something, you have to be there. It's a crazy place, and like any city, there are great places to eat and party. But it can get too crazy — and I'm lucky I have my beach house to escape to.'

Renan is retired from the top forty-five now. I was talking to him at the Nova Schin Pro in Inbituba, the second-last event on the World Championship Tour. He was doing some reporting for Sport TV in Brazil. Only the week before, he had won a 6 Star World Qualifying Series event against guys half his age. People couldn't believe it. The fact that he won this is testimony to every Brazilian surfer, whose whole life revolves around the saying 'Where there is a will, there is a way!'

## JUNGLE FEVER

On the outskirts of Sao Paulo, over lush green mountains and past the small fishing villages, are endless beaches. The scene is beautiful. Birds of paradise fly between the swaying green palms; you can hear monkeys and the beat of the bongo drums from the community hall on the beach where locals are practising capoeira. Life breathes and beats all around you. We were in Ubatuba, the coastal retreat for the surfers of Sao Paulo.

'There are eighty-five beaches here and all have surf,' boasted surfer/shaper Zecao, our host for the next few days. At thirty-eight years old, Zecao is a living legend. A second-generation surfer and Brazil's first touring professional, everywhere he goes Zecao is received with trademark double shakas. Though proud of his country, he also acknowledges the bitter taste of Third World corruption through his ever-present humour.

'The cops stop you all the time,' he said as we drove past a checkpoint on our way to surf. 'They only want money.' Later that day I told him how the Portuguese actually were the first to discover Australia, but unlike when they discovered Brazil, declined to set up a colony, sailing past the barren desert of Western Australia. His reaction was emphatic: 'You are lucky!'

Zecao described the beaches and coastline of Ubatuba like one would an epic girlfriend, drawing curves with his hands as we drove the twenty minutes north, past the few police roadblocks for our first surf check.

The scenery was very arousing. Massively steep mountains clothed in the green of the jungle met suddenly with the ocean, dropping off and often rising again to form many magnificent islands. 'There are many animals here,' stated Zecao proudly. 'We have small tigers [leopards], sloths, monkeys. Some Indians too!' (The native

Indians make up less than 1 per cent of the population and usually dwell in the jungles of the Amazon.) This was awesome. Kind of like the Brazil you pictured as a grommet: beach meets Amazon. But it was missing the one element that brings most people to Brazil — beautiful women. So it was off to Florianopolis to finish the story.

## FLORI

Getting there was going to be hard. 'How you going?' Mick Fanning had texted for the fourth time as I made my way down what we call 'death highway' by myself towards the WCT event in Florianopolis. It's a narrow highway full of swerve-inspiring potholes, crazy Mack trucks overtaking each other on blind corners and little cars getting run off the road. In Brazil, it is not against the law to drink drive. When you consider that, and also take into account the bad state of the roads and Brazilians' natural recklessness, it is not surprising to learn that 80,000 people die each year on Brazil's roads. It is a scary statistic that exemplifies how the Brazilian passion for life outweighs their fear of death. I was worried, but I ended up getting there in one piece.

Florianopolis, or 'Flori' as they call it, is actually an island made up mainly of sand. There are long beaches everywhere, littered with good banks. The human smorgasboard is made up of mainly rich and middle-class residents — and lots of hot girls! Therefore it's generally a safe and alluring place for the travelling surfer. But if you want to find trouble, it is never too far away — parties and drugs are endemic.

It's pretty easy to lead a laidback existence here: go to the beach in the afternoon, relax in the sun, wash off the hangover in the warm water, then do it all over again. It's kind of how people live here.

Well, most, but not everyone.

## THROUGH NECO'S EYES

I was sitting with Neco Padaratz, Brazil's favourite surfing son, on his home beach at Florianopolis. The men all around us were wearing their Speedos, playing batball on the beach and courting the girls by displaying their physical prowess while the girls flirted back by showing their own prowess — their beautiful bodies. Beyond them, the waves rolled in. And roll is all they do. There are little reef breaks here, but very few points; only miles of beach breaks. It's made being a professional surfer hard for people like Neco. He explained it to me.

'We have a lot of people here in Brazil working hard to make something of themselves. You have to go and if you don't go, watch out! Because someone will knock you over. Surfing in Brazil is intense. It's not like in most countries where you take your turn and relax with the ocean. Brazilians are incredibly full on. If someone gets the inside of you, it's their wave — and they'll go, yelling and screaming all the way. Intensity is in their blood. It's not just the way they live, but also the way they survive.

'When everybody thinks of Brazil,' said Neco, 'they think of carnival, they think of women, they think of the party. That's all they see. But there is the other side. There is tragedy, there is violence. It's unknown and it's sad that people can make such a beautiful land become such a horrible place.'

To make something of yourself in Brazil, you've got to do it by being more passionate and more competitive than anyone else. Adversity is par for the Brazilian course — and to rise above it takes incredible determination.

'When you live in Brazil, you are subject to everything,' said Neco. 'You really need the money and you need to work but there is so much corruption.'

In a country where you are either really rich or really poor, the Padaratz family were among the lucky ones. They grew up inland at a place called Blumenau before moving to Florianopolis, the wealthy cosmopolitan island in the south of Brazil. 'We just went down to the ocean one day,' said Neco. 'And for some reason, we never came back.'

He learned to surf on the many beach breaks around Florianopolis. It was a good training ground. He also had the advantage of having as an older brother Flavio Padaratz — the most successful surfer to come out of Brazil, who now runs the WCT event there and who still rips, despite being on the wrong side of forty!

The main criticism of Brazilian surfers is that they are supreme small wave surfers, but lack the power and technique to surf properly when the waves are perfect. This is because of the waves — or lack of waves — that they have in their homeland, which means that their technique favours short, flat turns. But it's not just the waves that make professional surfing on the world stage hard for Brazilians; there are also the cultural differences.

'It's really hard to be respected as a surfer today in Brazil,' said Neco, who actually moved to Australia in 1994 to learn English and develop his surfing. 'It's not easy to get money and then when you get it, you have to prove you are determined and that you want to fight. In Brazil our money is not worth much and we have big economic problems. A lot of the surfers don't speak English because we are such a poor country and it's difficult to get educated. To send them out to the world and say "Be a pro surfer" is really tough. We need to stick together, and the more Brazilians that travel, the more powerful we can be.'

The thought of that sends a shiver down the spine. Anyone who has travelled and come across Brazilians is easily frustrated by their lack of etiquette in the water. They are intensely competitive everywhere they go. They are loud, and dominate line-ups. Unfortunately, to some extent they do carry their culture of 'run over or be run over' around the world. Every sport has rules and in Brazil, you use them to be the best. It's why their soccer players collapse theatrically when they're tackled and why their surfers snake you. They are not just trying to be better, but doing what's inculcated in them: survival.

Brazilian people show their emotions like no other people. The first time I ever went to Brazil was in 1994. It was for the World Amateur Titles in Rio and we arrived to see a country draped in black. It was the day Ayrton Senna died and the Brazilian president had declared a day of mourning. I vividly remember arriving at my hotel and seeing a seventeen-year-old Neco Padaratz crying in the lift.

It was a typical display of passion for Neco's country. 'I carry my flag with me on everything. My bags, my board covers. Not just because I'm Brazilian and it's in my blood, but also to say, "Look, I'm from far away, man — and I fought all my life to try and be something." Whether I win or lose, I need to carry that message,' he explained.

Though surfing is starting to gain massive support in Brazil, it is still a long way behind football. On every street corner, kids play soccer; on a fresh pitch in a rich suburb, or on a dirt paddock in a *favela*. These are the people who, like Neco, are trying to make something of themselves, trying to break out of the *favela* and make a life. It has been proven by people before them that with hard work it is possible; people who play with more passion and intensity than the next guy can rise above their squalor. On the soccer pitch and in the surf, everybody can be a winner.

'I train every day and sweat every day to make something of my life. If I spend every energy inside me to surf, people can respect that. You have to do something for the will — and never give up. I'm helping my kid a lot more too. He is getting big and surfing already.' Neco had the proudest expression on his face as he pointed to the tattoo of his son on his arm.

'I want him to know that when I come back from overseas, I come back as a professional surfer and that he can respect that because I trained so hard to be where I am now. I do that because there is a kid who depends on my dream of being something. People need to know why I scream and sometimes go crazy. Every time I win a heat, it's another bottle of milk that I can buy for him, so there is a lot of reason for it. I am really passionate about the sport that I do. It's my everything; it is my breathing. It will give him some direction, so I cannot surrender. I WILL be something so that he can be something too.'

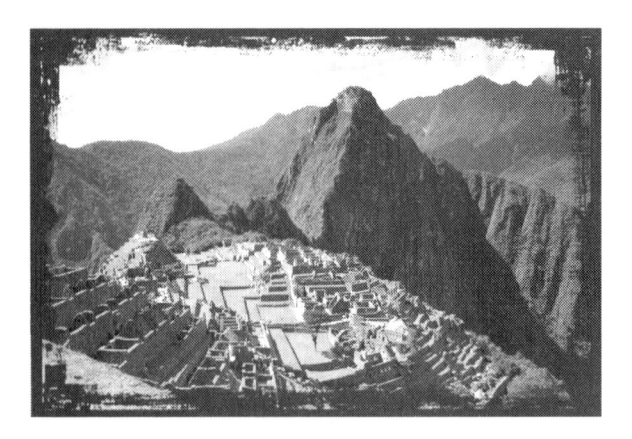

# THE SANDS OF ALL TIME
PERU

Dave Rastovich rose from his two-hour daily ritual of meditation and yoga exhilarated. 'I can't wait for tomorrow. I can't wait for Chicama, I can't wait for Machu Picchu, I can't wait for the next breath.' His genuine excitement was palpable.

In front of him, the Pacific Ocean gave life to all the senses. We watched sea birds mingle with pelicans, chasing tuna, chasing anchovies. The desert earth hurt our feet. The landscape was dead, lifeless and unforgiving: a narrow corridor, a void of death. To our back were the Andean mountains, loaded with geographical wonders and Inca mysteries. It was a land of contrasting extremities. We were in a place like no other.

## LEARNING LIMA

'When the Spanish conquered the Incas in 1532,' said Magoo de la Rosa, Peruvian surfing champion, 'they asked them where the best place on the coast was to build a city.' He laughed with an intense energy possessed by most South Americans — a welcoming, contagious laugh that knows no tomorrow. 'The Incas told them to come here — to Lima.' He cracked up, pointing to the depressing and dry landscape around his nation's capital. 'Because they knew it was the worst place in Peru!'

We arrived in Lima on flight AR1365 via Auckland and Buenos Aires. Even in the heat of the day, the desert coast around Lima seemed to sleep under a resident blanket of haze. There are no bright colours there, just monotones of sandy brown and greys that I'd only seen in Salvador Dali paintings; endless dunes and grey skies.

'This is bizarre,' piped up Dave Rastovich (Rasta), who admitted to having previously visited in his dreams. 'It's so surreal. I reckon this is what the moon looks like.' Rasta's a man who appreciates adventures and examines everything through a spiritual lens. He was a good partner to have on the trip because his appreciation and enthusiasm know no bounds.

When we arrived in the southern town of San Bartolo, the scene was magical. Spanish churches and Inca shadows lingered on the desert shores. People of mixed descent played in the ocean; some surfing, some swimming, and some eating. The cultures of Peru don't clash; they dance in the fading orange and celebrate their past. The people are open and welcoming and you feel a part of their lives as soon as you meet them.

'Here is Alto Pico,' said Magoo's best friend, Oscar. He described the surrounding coastline to us while the desert sand tested his trusty four-wheel drive. 'It's a famous big wave spot here in Peru. There is a point break here also ... and here ... and there.' He pointed as he laughed. 'Peru is full of point breaks.'

The famous Pan Pacific Highway slithers along the entire Peruvian coastline, mostly in view of the ocean. Many travellers are lured by its path. While you can see the waves from the highway, it's necessary to take the small bumpy roads into tiny fishing villages to check the surf. We surfed many of these places in the first few days of our trip. For example, Senoritas is a rippable left-hander with another bommie-type right-hander that offered plenty of raw power and open face, although both were a little fat. Despite the deep ocean trench just 100 kilometres off the coast, and the Andean mountains that rise to 7000 metres, only 100 kilometres inland, the coastline seems to linger in the shallows as if scared to get its rocks in the cold water. The waves are strong, but due to this gradual gradient, they don't barrel or break with too much authority. They are long, but not fast. They dribble instead of spit, but roll in with an accommodating rhythm.

From the line-up you see an incredible array of contrasts. You really feel as if you are in another world. We watched fish jumping around everywhere; chasing, being chased. It's a comfortable feeling watching the shark-less ocean come alive. In one spot offshore from Lima there is a place where the annual catch of anchovies is enough to feed six million people per year. Pelicans were everywhere — trimming their darker feathers confidently across the surface of the ocean, but rarely crossing land. The shoreline is like a border to another world — and anything that crosses it, usually dies. There is no life there. It is the driest desert coast in the world. No colours, no animals, no trees; not even a blade of grass. The desert sucks the life out of any bird drawn inland, usually within a few hours.

'Okay,' announced Oscar grandly as we entered Marky's Hotel where we were staying. 'Tomorrow we go to the mountains. I have looked on the Internet and there is no swell for one week. *Vamanos!*' In Spanish the word means, 'Let's go', and when you are in a country that doesn't know how to pull back, you soon learn it.

## CUZCO

The short flight from Lima to Cuzco was breathtaking. The grey of the desert coast had receded into a brilliant blue sky as mountains, often snow-capped, raced us to 9000 metres. Life flooded back. We were ascending into the Andes, a place where clouds gather thick with mystery, and where for one civilisation — the Incas — life began.

The founder of the city was Wira Cocha. Mythological stories have passed down the tale of a white man who arrived at Lake Titicaca, which borders Peru and Bolivia, after a great drought killed many of the mountain villagers around AD 1100. He taught the survivors about western civilisation, and then quickly vanished back to whence he came. The survivors founded Cuzco as their religious base and, under Wira Cocha's instructions, built a city in the shape of a puma, their god of strength. For three centuries the people flourished, building intricate roadworks to connect them to an empire that, by the Spanish conquest in 1532, had grown to thirteen million people and covered most of South America. They were called the Incas — and we were arriving at what they called 'the navel of the world'.

'You have to be careful,' warned Oscar as we climbed through the city of Cuzco to the sacred ruins of Saqsaywaman — the puma's head. 'This is the highest concentrated energy source on earth.' The ruins stood watchful over the city. The stones, some weighing 130 tonnes, were cut perfectly. They zigzagged across the higher plane for 100 metres giving shape to the puma's teeth, then mouth, then head, until the neck fell down the mountain to find the puma's body. From the top you could see the heart (the city square), the reproductive organs (the church), the body and the tail.

There is no need for cement or mortar between the stones; they are an exact fit. Some have up to ten angles on them with gaps that couldn't accommodate the thinnest of razor blades. The walls are built with seven-degree angles and from stones of asymmetrical shapes so that when the turbulent land quaked, the stones could be drawn into each other, making the walls stronger. This was no backward civilisation.

As we climbed higher and the air got thinner, we walked into what our guide informed us was the energy centre. Enclosed in what had formerly been a nine-metre-high gold-plated circle, now reduced to a gold-less three feet, was the puma's eye.

'I got to go,' said Rasta, freaking out. He seeks solitude like the thirsty crave water. While he went off to meditate, I was overdosing on a strange sensation. I found myself running from wall to wall, dancing and floating like a butterfly. I was encouraged to sit cross-legged in a circle and to put my hands within an inch of each other. They started to burn up as if they were attempting to make fire. I closed my eyes and my body seemed to float inches above the dirt. It was intense. Oscar, who is usually all fun and games, grabbed me and told me his life story, hugging me and opening up a dam of emotion as if he was intoxicated. Where was Rasta? I needed his solitude. I ran from the ring, oblivious to the lack of oxygen in my muscles and lungs. I looked over the city of Cuzco. It was about a kilometre below me, enveloped by a mammoth mountain and river. I said hello to the puma.

'This is like some fantasy world,' said Rasta. 'It doesn't feel real. Imagine the energy here ...' He floated off to harness the energy and meditate somewhere else as I became increasingly drunk on the Inca and Andean history. Eighty million years ago, the Andes sat at the bottom of the ocean. Fossils of conch shells and other fish mingle with the remnants of Inca history, highlighting the wonders of nature's extremities.

'The puma's head was built in 1430,' said our guide. I forgot he was there. 'It was finished in 1470 by 200,000 people. They moved the rocks on trees that had small stones underneath them, acting as rollers.' I thought of my own research — how traces of cocaine had been found in mummified tombs in ancient Egypt dating back to 2000 BC (cocaine originated in Peru). The connections and parallels between the Peruvians, the people of Easter Island, Egyptians, Central Americans and Polynesians are dazzling. Wira Cocha, who sailed from the west to teach the Incas, is also found in Polynesian mythology, where he is known as Maui. He is also known as Viracocha in other distant places. My mind raced and I finally laughed. We hadn't even gone to Machu Picchu yet and I was already sinking into the biggest natural hangover of my life.

Two old ladies draped in traditional Incan dress — bright red dresses and with their hair in long pigtails — sat next to me in the plaza of Cuzco. For their age, they were beautiful. Spanish culture surrounded us, intertwined, and built on — like most of the city — Inca stonework. The Spanish demolished many buildings after their conquest. They stripped the city and turned it upside down like a pair of jeans and shook all the gold out of its pockets. I imagined the Spaniards riding over the hills, equipped with horses, weapons and disease; I imagined what a city plated in gold would look like. The city had suffered two earthquakes since the Spaniards rode over those hills and although the Spanish-built churches have crumbled, the Incan foundations remain — as do the spirits of those who built them.

I wondered what the ladies were talking about. They talked so peacefully and sparingly, often enjoying minutes of silence together. Like the Incan legacy, time doesn't matter to them anymore. They just sit and watch. I sat with them for two hours and practised my Spanish. It was a highlight.

## THE CITY IN THE SKY

'*Esta bien?*' asked the conductor as he walked through the train carriage. 'Is everything okay?' Like a ship sailing against the forces of nature, the train from Cuzco to Machu Picchu fought its way through the rugged terrain. We had changed course, going backwards and forwards a couple of times, and everyone had lost their sense of direction. Powered by its own momentum, the train climbed like a roller coaster in slow motion, and then back down the other side in its ritual dance with the mountains. The dance wasn't lost on the train driver who smiled proudly at his method of conquering the ancient landscape.

American Hiram Bingham discovered Machu Picchu, the 'lost city of the Incas', in 1911. What he found under the dense shrub was a city in the shape of a condor — a tribute to the Incan god of wisdom — flying high above an intensely jagged landscape. As we journeyed higher, the mountains became steeply vertical, falling into deep, shadowed valleys with barely enough room for the gushing river to escape its own claustrophobia. After an hour and a half of vertical climbing, we reached the top of Huancho Picchu, the adjacent mountain to Machu Picchu. 'We're so used to seeing ground in front of us,' pondered Jon Frank, our photographer. 'Look,' he said pointing with his outstretched arm, 'there's nothing but air.' And so we sat for two hours in space and time and never talked about life so clearly and simply.

Later I found Rasta — an even harder task — meditating on top of a once-lonely rock halfway up the condor's wing. The clouds gathered menacingly below us: we were so high (2900 metres above sea level) that the cloud enveloped us. It was like an Inca ghost telling us it was closing time. 'This has been one of the best days of my life,' he admitted.

## CHICAMA

'Harvey is the best surfer in Peru,' said Tonio, a friend we had gathered along the way. We had gone back to the desert coast and Tonio was our driver for the trip up to Chicama, which possessed the world's longest wave. Peruvians often have friends who are the best at something, or at least the adjective is used liberally. I had already heard of twenty world champions at twelve different sports. Oddly enough, the one confirmed sighting was of the World Champion Man and Dog surfing team. We barbecued at his house in San Bartolo and he proudly showed me the trophy and brought out a photo of him and his dog surfing in Hawaii. And if that didn't prove it, he ordered his dog to fetch me a beer — which it did.

In Tonio's car, we were back on the long winding road of the Pan Pacific Highway, making the greatly anticipated journey to Chicama. We listened to plenty of reggae on the trip up, Peru's favourite sound. It's amazing what effect music can have on you when you have been away from it for a while. But what we were experiencing was something more, an enhanced sensation. We pulled over in the failing light to camp out at Playa Grande (Big Beach) and started dancing in the car and then nude swimming in the ocean — relaxed and floating around.

'When you come down from the altitude the increased oxygen makes you feel like you're on cocaine,' offered Tonio. Well that made sense.

We chewed each other's ears off and slept under the stars that night, the haze we had once despised as our only blanket. We awoke in the morning to the sound of small waves and to the smell of salt water and dead animals. We were back. Bones and carcasses lay everywhere, victims of the desert.

'*Cuando las olas son grandes.*' My Spanish was enjoying its first real workout with local surfer, Jesus, as we arrived at Chicama. He told me of the four-kilometre wave that fans perfectly from point to pier and how he is one of the few locals who lives and surfs there. Most of the locals borrow boards from tourists, as they cannot afford their own. He described the wave to me, with dancing arms and double shakas and I enjoyed the universal happiness of surfers. At three foot, Chicama rocked my world, and unlike most of the waves we had seen, the resident offshore wind ensured tubes. They spin as consistently as the windmill on the overlooking cliff that provides the small town's electricity. Chicama is definitely one of surfing's natural wonders. We surfed it for hours and rode the longest waves of our lives.

The next morning Jesus declared, 'Today you must go to Pacasmayo. You'll have big waves over there.'

At first, we could barely see Pacasmayo through the omnipresent haze. It was yet another small fishing village whose immediate impact was lost on us. We moved slowly and I didn't see Rasta until I was paddling twenty metres from him. 'It's pumping,' he yelled between spirited gulps of fog. 'I just got a perfect section in a row for about fifteen turns. This place is amazing!'

And it was. It was one of those waves you can't see the end of. You can really tune your surfing and your board here in Peru. If you butcher one section, there'll be twenty more just like it. Where you want to surf the wave and how you want to surf it is up to you. And as usual, there were no locals, just a Pommy and a Kiwi backpacker.

I left the long point break with a goal scored: I had ridden the longest wave of my life, and it wasn't at Chicama as I had expected. I could have set the record at any one of twenty different places.

Like the long point breaks and magnificent landscapes, there is something mysterious and timeless about Peru. You go there with a vision that can fit inside your head, and leave with knowledge of a place that is more infinite than the universe. It opens your world to the extremes of nature and human mystery. It's an intellectual and geographical phenomenon. There are few trees in the country, but their roots seem to go on forever. I thought about the world's longest left, the world's driest desert coast, and the world's second greatest mountain range — and the Incas. And just when I thought I was starting to understand it, I met someone else.

## GODS OF THE SEA

'Modern surfing may have started in Hawaii, but when did surfing really begin?' wondered Molars, whose mouth opened into an enormous smile, revealing the origin of his nickname. But he was talking about the origins of surfing — a subject as hot as the surrounding desert for any Peruvian surfer. Their ancestors built pyramids, conquered most of South America, mastered the elements — and may just have been the first people to experience the sensation of riding a wave.

It is a huge question — who first rode the waves — and I was starting to discover that the answer has lain buried in the sandy coastal desert of Peru for centuries. Pre-Incan ceramics dating back to 600 BC show the first evidence, to date, of wave riding. This newfound proof takes the origins of wave riding back at least 2300 years. That's 700 years before Hawaii was even settled. And many people in Peru, a nation already graced with historic mystery, believe it could go back even further.

'Why not?' asked Roberto Meza Vallue. He held a small replica of the original 'surfboards' to the light, pausing to examine the surfboard-like rocker as if it were his own new shape. At full size, the reed-woven vessels — called *totoras* — were between nine to fifteen feet in length and around 60 centimetres wide. They consisted of two cylindrical sections, like a tightly-jointed catamaran, and a nose that thinned out into a wild-rockered surfboard simulation. Resembling a cross between a surfboard and a wave ski, they seem to unite necessity and recreation in one — fishing and surfing. And that's exactly what they were used for.

'It is pre-Inca, pre-Christian — pre-everything,' explained Roberto with a twinkle of pride. Like his country, his olive skin and wild surfer's hair have been created by a combination of Indian and Spanish blood. A former champion and big wave specialist, Roberto is helping research a book on the history of surfing in Peru — a story that is set to rock the surfing world.

'Before the Incas started conquering most of South America between the twelfth and sixteenth century, Peru was made up of small fishing communities,' said Roberto. The oldest remains of civilisation are from about 10,000 BC from Cultura Paiján. The people probably came by walking from the North Bering Strait. Coming to the driest desert in the world, these small Peruvian tribes managed to survive with the help of the ocean. The only water from the Andes flows west to the Amazon. With no rain, few rivers and an arid soil, on which it is almost impossible to cultivate plants, these tribes relied on the ocean for survival. And this is how they started wave riding.

'Modern surfing may have started in Hawaii,' said Roberto. 'But when did wave riding start? We Peruvians say that the *totoras* were the first surfing instruments of the world.' Hidden in the ancient sands of Peru are thousands of ceramics that depict these *totora* sea horses — and people riding waves on them.

'They were used for fishing,' said Javier Fernandez, editor of *Tablista*, Peru's surfing magazine. He also keeps a small model in his downtown Lima office. When we spoke, he was wearing a Duke Kahanamoku shirt and a nervous grin, and his excitement was frustrated by his limited English. 'There are not many channels in Peru,' he explained. 'So they would kneel down and paddle them through the surf to fish in deeper waters. When they came in at the end of the day they would stand up on the surfboard and ride the wave in. It was important for them to teach the young ones wave skills as well, so they shaped smaller *totoras*, with three circular components of thatched reed, so that the young ones could practise with more stability before progressing on to the more traditional ones.'

One day I walked through the National Museum of Ceramic Art in Lima. It was one of my first steps in a long voyage of discovery. The potteries in the museum were full of surfing depictions. The ocean was the Peruvian people's life and wave riding was a big part of it. This was the biggest thing that stood out to me — Peru was a surfing culture.

Testimonies from locals, as well as ceramics dating back 1200 years, tell of a smaller version of the instruments, which were paddled like today's surfboards. These scaled-down versions, perhaps six foot eight in length, were designed for days when the surf was big and the larger *totoras* found it difficult to get out to the deep waters for fishing. The craftsmanship of these instruments reveals an incredibly evolved knowledge of waves and an insight into surfboard design that rivals those of today's most advanced minds.

'For sure they were into surfing,' said Magoo de la Rosa Toro, a seven-time Peruvian surfing champion, who has enough gold on his trophy cabinet to rival the Incan royal family. At thirty-six, Magoo's energy and passion for surfing is unrivalled. So too is his passion for history. His backyard houses the beginnings of a surfboard museum, including the *totoras*, and we walked through it like it was the Garden of Eden. 'Look at the *totoras*,' he said, pushing aside the rare balsa wood surfboard. 'They have perfect rocker — they were much better designed for surfing than fishing.'

Later that week, we watched two locals paddle out on the *totoras* at Huanchaco. Huanchaco is the traditional birthplace and current stable of today's sea horses. The surfers turned around and stood up, manoeuvred with their oar towards the shore, and rode the waves effortlessly and naturally. 'They are hard to ride,' admitted Magoo. 'You can't turn them but you can go straight. You have to turn with the oar — that's like their fin.'

The main thing I noticed — which is common to all surfers — was the smiles on their faces. 'There's no way they just used them for fishing,' said Magoo. 'Look at them. Look how happy he is. Who can catch just one wave and come in?' He hungrily ate a pile of *ceviche*, the traditional dish of Peru. 'You can taste the food in Peru — but you cannot taste the history.'

Archaeologists and historians believe that both the high chiefs and the common people used the *totoras* for competitions in wave riding and paddling events — and that these were common occurrences. However, their writings must rely only on physical facts, such as the ceramics and the Spanish chronicles written after the conquest in 1532. Very little is known and so much is yet to be discovered; the locals are not the only ones who are theorising.

'This is just the earliest evidence to date,' said Maria, who is writing a book with the help of Magoo and Roberto. 'I think the *totoras* are at least 5000 years old. They have just found remains of fishing nets that date from that time.' She paused, allowing obvious questions to arise. 'Where do you catch bigger fish, or where do you use fishing nets? Further out. How do you get there? With a boat. What is the only boat used by the pre-Incas? The *totoras*. How do you get in? Catch waves.' I remembered the faces of those two surfers ecstatic riding waves on the *totoras*. 'Just because the ceramic era didn't start till later doesn't mean they were not surfing before then.'

The ceramic era started in Peru around 1000 BC. As there is no written record from the Incas or their ancestors prior to 1532, Peruvian history has generally been written by the Spanish conquistadors.

'I was in Huanchaco five years ago,' said Adolfo Valderrama Bielich, who perhaps offered the most detailed opinion on the subject. He is a 46-year-old economist, teacher and surfer; an intellectual who wears Coke bottles as spectacles and rides surfboards as high on the face as the pants that choked his throat. An athlete and an intellectual, he pronounced ancient languages and spoke of long-ago cultures with practised ease.

'It was a good day for surfing,' he continued. 'I spoke to an old indigenous fisherman. We were watching the surfers and he was saying, "I remember doing that when I was a child." He told me how his father also used to speak of riding the waves when he was young. This is especially important because it shows that surfing was done when they were kids, or for a ceremony. Otherwise it was irresponsible. Just like today, people have jobs and chores that take priority; in those days theirs was to fish. They say only a surfer knows the feeling. When I met that old man, he could still feel it!'

Adolfo had been studying the history of the *totoras* from 1992 to '96, following the studies of Don Guillermo Wiesse and Fortunato Quezada Lagarrigue. He had initially agreed with Wiesse and had concluded that the main purpose of the *totoras* was for fishing. 'But after that day,' said Adolfo, 'after listening to that old man at Huanchaco, I knew there was another explanation. Sure, the main purpose was to fish. But the vessels were also used for wave riding.

'The *totoras* only have a life span of sixty days,' he pointed to his own surfboard, yellow with age, and I imagined the reeds softening and losing their drive. 'After that period they would pass them down to the kids to develop their ocean skills. They were the ones who surfed day in, day out. There were also special *totoras* made for competitions where the elders could show their skills.

'It is also important to note that the fishing net remains from the *hombre de parcas* — 'man of fates', the people of 6800 BC — are the earliest evidence of net fishing in the world today. It shows the level of civilisation these people had and their affinity with the ocean. Later pictures on the pyramids and the ceramics confirm their existence, as well as the Spanish chronicles.'

When the Spanish conquistadors arrived in northern Peru in 1528, they observed something they had never before witnessed — surfing. One wordsmith made this poetic entry in his ship's log:

> '... A native gliding over the ocean on what seemed to be graceful sea horses. They cut through the water, advancing with their long necks propelled forward with an easy rhythm of grace and beauty. Indeed a beautiful sight to behold, as they dance over the swells, they return with the waves and the foam, as carefree as musical notes in a pagan celebration. At times they seem totally lost among the breakers, only to reappear as if engaged in a game with the sea. As sunset roars, they return toward shore for their last ride. A lovely sight in the fresh and golden sunlight. Their mounts like spirited stallions, now tremble, then rear and finally race toward shore, [and] those golden bare chested men staying barely in front of the tumbling foam seem to be "gods of the Sea"'.

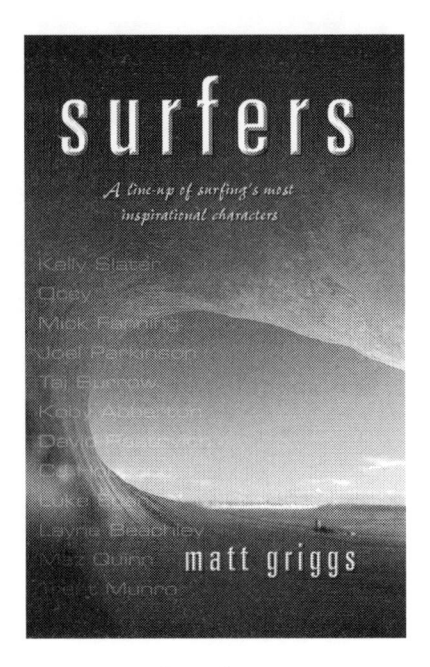

## Surfers

MATT GRIGGS

A line-up of surfing's most inspirational characters

Jump in the V8s of Mick Fanning, Joel Parkinson and Dean Morrison in Coolangatta. Stroke into a set at Waimea Bay with Kieren Perrow. Go on a spiritual adventure with David Rastovich in Peru. Enjoy a country beer with Trent Munro at Scotts Head. Learn of Koby Abberton's hard — and softer — side at Maroubra. Encounter the surfing culture of Brazil and New Zealand with Neco Padaratz and Maz Quinn. Survive a near-death experience at G-land with Luke Egan. Get inside the creative minds of Oscar Wright and photographer Jon Frank. Relive the ten-year surfing odyssey of Peter Troy and enjoy the youthful exploits of Luke Munro. Cheer one of the world's least accomplished professional surfers, Wade Glasscock, and admire the world's best, Kelly Slater. And wonder at Taj Burrow's legendary prowess with the ladies ...

In *Surfers*, former professional surfer, *Tracks* writer and current international team pit boss, Matt Griggs, gives an insider's view of a line-up of surfing's most interesting and unique characters. At turns funny and sad but always inspiring, it lifts the lid on one of the world's most dynamic, enigmatic and mysterious sports.